Atlas of CSF Cytology

Harald Kluge
Valentin Wieczorek †
Ernst Linke
Klaus Zimmermann
Stefan Isenmann
Otto W. Witte

With contributions by

M. Gajda
H. Guhlmann
M. Kiehntopf
M. M. Kluska
H.-J. Kuehn
R. Lehmitz

M. Roskos
E. Schulze
E. Sindern
E. Taub
M. Wick

304 illustrations

Georg Thieme Verlag
Stuttgart · New York

IV

Library of Congress Cataloging-in-Publication Data

Atlas der praktischen Liquorzytologie. English.
Atlas of CSF cytology / editors, Harald Kluge ... [et al.] ; with
contributions by M. Gajda ... [et al.].
  p. ; cm.
Includes bibliographical references and index.
ISBN 3-13-143161-X (GTV : alk. paper)
ISBN 1-58890-546-2 (GTV : alk. paper)
ISBN (invalid) 3-13-143161-5 (TNY : alk. paper)
ISBN (invalid) 1-58890-546-8 (TNY : alk. paper) 1. Cerebrospinal
fluid–Atlases. 2. Cytodiagnosis–Atlases. I. Kluge, Harald. II. Title.
[DNLM: 1. Cerebrospinal Fluid–cytology–Atlases. QY 17 A8745a
2007a].
RB55.A85 2007
612.8′042–dc22

2006032048

This book is an authorized and revised translation of the German
edition published and copyrighted 2005 by Georg Thieme Verlag,
Stuttgart, Germany. Title of the German edition: Atlas der praktischen Liquorzytologie.

Translator: Ethan Taub, MD, Zurich, Switzerland

The authors welcome comments, suggestions, and submissions of
additional illustrations (rare cytological images). Please, send cor-
respondence to
Prof. Stefan Isenmann
Department of Neurology
Friedrich-Schiller-University Jena
Erlanger Allee 101
07747 Jena
Germany
Email: stefan.isenmann@med.uni-jena.de

© 2007 Georg Thieme Verlag,
Rüdigerstraße 14, 70469 Stuttgart, Germany
http://www.thieme.de
Thieme New York, 333 Seventh Avenue,
New York, NY 10001, USA
http://www.thieme.com

Cover illustration: Martina Berge, Erbach, Germany

Typesetting by Sommer Druck, Feuchtwangen
Printed in Germany by Appl · Aprinta, Wemding

ISBN-10: 3-13-143161-X (GTV)
ISBN-13: 978-3-13-143161-5 (GTV)
ISBN-10: 1-58890-546-2 (TNY)
ISBN-13: 978-1-58890-546-8 (TNY)   1 2 3 4 5 6

Important note: Medicine is an ever-changing science undergoing
continual development. Research and clinical experience are con-
tinually expanding our knowledge, in particular our knowledge of
proper treatment and drug therapy. Insofar as this book mentions
any dosage or application, readers may rest assured that the authors, editors, and publishers have made every effort to ensure that
such references are in accordance with **the state of knowledge at
the time of production of the book.**
Nevertheless, this does not involve, imply, or express any guarantee
or responsibility on the part of the publishers in respect to any dosage instructions and forms of applications stated in the book. **Every
user is requested to examine carefully** the manufacturers' leaflets
accompanying each drug and to check, if necessary in consultation
with a physician or specialist, whether the dosage schedules mentioned therein or the contraindications stated by the manufacturers differ from the statements made in the present book. Such
examination is particularly important with drugs that are either
rarely used or have been newly released on the market. Every dosage schedule or every form of application used is entirely at the
user's own risk and responsibility. The authors and publishers re-
quest every user to report to the publishers any discrepancies or in-
accuracies noticed.

Addresses

Mieczyslaw Gajda, MD
Institute of Pathology
University Hospital Jena
Jena, Germany

Hanno Guhlmann, MD
Jena, Germany

Stefan Isenmann, MD
Professor of Neurology
Supervising Physician, CSF Diagnostics
Department of Neurology
University Hospital Jena
Jena, Germany

Michael Kiehntopf, MD
Institute of Clinical Chemistry and CSF Diagnostic
Studies
University Hospital Jena
Jena, Germany

Harald Kluge, MD
Former Professor and Head of the Central CSF
Laboratory
Faculty of Medicine and Institute of Clinical Chemistry
University of Jena
Jena, Germany

Martin Marian Kluska, MD
Institute of Anatomy and Cytology
University Clinic Heidelberg
Heidelberg, Germany

Hans-Juergen Kuehn, MD
Head of Section for CSF Diagnostic Studies
Clinical Chemistry and Molecular Diagnostic Testing
Institute for Laboratory Medicine
University Clinic Leipzig
Leipzig, Germany

Reinhard Lehmitz, MD
Central CSF Laboratory
Center of Neurology
University Clinic Rostock
Rostock, Germany

Ernst Linke, MD
Former Head of Central Laboratory
Currently Scientific supervisor of Central CSF
Laboratory
Asklepios Hospital
Stadtroda, Germany

Martin Roskos, MD
Private Practice
Jena, Germany

Eberhard Schulze, MD
Institute of Pathology
University Hospital Jena
Jena, Germany

Eckhardt Sindern, MD
Professor of Neurology
Ev. Diakoniewerk Friederikenstift Hospital
Hanover, Germany

Ethan Taub, MD
Diplomate of the American Board of Neurological
Surgery
Klinik Im Park
Zurich, Switzerland

Manfred Wick, MD
Institute of Clinical Chemistry
Department of Protein Chemistry and
Immunochemistry
University Hospital Munich
Munich, Germany

Valentin Wieczorek †
Professor emeritus
Faculty of Medicine
Hans Berger Hospital of Neurology
University of Jena
Jena, Germany

O. W. Witte, MD
Professor of Neurology
Head of Hans Berger Hospital of Neurology
University of Jena
Jena, Germany

Klaus Zimmermann, MD
Head of Section for CSF Diagnostic Studies
Medical Laboratory Dresden/Elsterwerda
Laboratory Dr. Pontek/Dr. Bochmann
Dresden, Germany

Foreword

by the German Society for the Diagnostic Study of the Cerebrospinal Fluid and Clinical Neurochemistry

The importance of diagnostic study of the cerebrospinal fluid (CSF) is evident to all neurologists, neurosurgeons, psychiatrists, pediatricians, and internists, and to specialists in many other medical disciplines. Without CSF studies, a large number of clinical diagnoses could never be made or confirmed. Among all studies of this type, *cytological examination of the CSF* plays a central, indispensable role. Its proper performance demands considerable expertise, but it can nevertheless be accomplished relatively rapidly and inexpensively. The authors thus deserve all the more praise for preparing this comprehensive cytological atlas. This reference work illustrates CSF cytological findings with more than 300 beautifully and sharply reproduced color images obtained from *clinical* studies. The authors' detailed and authoritative explanations draw on the expertise they have gained over decades of experience in CSF cytology. This atlas thus makes an important contribution to quality assurance in CSF diagnosis and to the training and continuing education of clinical CSF cytologists and laboratory physicians.

Cologne, Germany

H.-F. Petereit
Secretary of the Society

Preface

This cytological atlas is the product of many years of experience in *practical* cerebrospinal fluid (CSF) cytology. It is designed to meet the need for a new, *comprehensive* atlas some 25 years after the most recent ones appeared and to make a contribution toward the optimization of CSF cellular diagnosis.

The range of possible findings in CSF cytological studies is very wide, and misdiagnoses are thus likely if the examiner lacks sufficient knowledge and experience. We have thus put special emphasis on the presentation of typical cytological pictures in the acute and remission phases of diseases of the central nervous system (CNS), as well as typical cytological changes over the course of treatment. Furthermore, we suggest appropriate immunocytological studies for further work-up in cases where the routine cytological examination of the CSF alone does not yield a sufficiently precise cytological diagnosis.

The spectrum of CSF cytological pictures is systematically organized in diagnostic categories, i.e., infectious and inflammatory diseases of the CNS, intracranial hemorrhage, traumatic and hypoxic-ischemic brain damage, and malignant processes with neoplastic meningitis (with reference to the World Health Organization classification of brain tumors, 2000). In each chapter, the images are preceded by a brief theoretical discussion.

We thank our readers for their attention and hope this atlas will help and encourage them in the everyday laboratory practice of CSF cytology and in comparative cytological research. We would be glad to receive suggestions as to how the book might be further improved. We would be especially grateful for submissions of additional illustrations or of cytological preparations showing uncommon but diagnostically important findings (rarities).

We thank Georg Thieme Verlag, and in particular Marion Ueckert, Ursula Biehl-Vatter, Korinna Engeli, and Gabriele Kuhn for their extensive help and advice during the preparation of this book. We are also grateful to Dr. Ethan Taub for his accurate and readable translation of the book into English.

Jena, Germany   *The editors and authors*

The authors report with sorrow that our co-author, Professor Valentin Wieczorek, one of the pioneering figures in the field of CSF cytology, died on July 15, 2005 as the original German edition of this atlas was going to print. The atlas represents a part of his life's work, and we regret that he did not live to see it published.

Table of Contents

1 Introduction 1

H. Kluge, V. Wieczorek, E. Linke, K. Zimmermann, O. W. Witte

Role of Practical (Classical) CSF
Cytological Examination in the Overall
Spectrum of CSF Diagnostic Studies ... 2

H. Kluge, V. Wieczorek, O. W. Witte, E. Linke,
K. Zimmermann, E. Taub, S. Isenmann

Diagnostic Use of Immunocytological
Phenotyping Techniques
in CSF Cytology 4

M. Wick, H. Kluge, E. Schulze, R. Lehmitz,
M. M. Kluska

Diagnostic Use of Flow Cytometry
in CSF Cytology 5

E. Sindern, M. Wick, M. Roskos, M. Kiehntopf,
H. Kluge

Proper Handling of CSF Specimens
Before Cytological Examination 7

H. Kluge, M. Roskos, E. Linke, V. Wieczorek,
E. Taub, S. Isenmann

Cell Preparation (Sedimentation)
and Staining 8

H. Kluge, M. Roskos, M. M. Kluska

The CSF Cytology Report: Consensus
Reporting Form of the German Society
for the Diagnostic Study of the
Cerebrospinal Fluid and Clinical
Neurochemistry for Use in On-Site
Round-Robin Tests 9

E. Linke, H. Kluge

2 Cell Populations in the Normal Cerebrospinal Fluid 13

H. Kluge, E. Linke, V. Wieczorek, K. Zimmermann, H.-J. Kuehn

Lymphocytes and Monocytes 13

Cells and Cell Clusters From the
Structures Enclosing the CSF Space ... 15

Lumbar Puncture Artifacts:
Bone Marrow Components,
Cartilage Cells, etc. 18

**3 Pathological CSF Cell Findings in Infectious and Inflammatory Diseases
    of the Central Nervous System** 21

V. Wieczorek, H. Kluge, E. Linke, R. Lehmitz, M. Gajda, H. Guhlmann, S. Isenmann

Granulocytes and Activated Forms
of the Lymphocytic Series 21

Cytological Findings in Infectious
and Inflammatory Diseases 25

**4 Pathological CSF Cell Findings in Intracranial Hemorrhage
    and Traumatic and Hypoxic-Ischemic Brain Injury** 45

H. Kluge, V. Wieczorek, O. W. Witte, E. Linke, K. Zimmermann, M. M. Kluska, S. Isenmann

On the Origin of Macrophages 47

5   Pathological CSF Cell Findings in Primary and Metastatic CNS Tumors, Malignant Lymphoma, and Leukemia 61

V. Wieczorek, H. Kluge, E. Linke, K. Zimmermann, H.-J. Kuehn, O. W. Witte, S. Isenmann

Fundamentals 61

Astrocytic Tumors 64

Ependymal Turmors 76

Tumors of the Chloroid Plexus 79

Ganglioglioma 81

Pineal Tumors 82

Medulloblastoma 84

Pituitary Adenoma 88

Mesenchymal, Non-Meningothelial Tumors 89

Germ Cell Tumors 94

Melanoma 96

Metastases 99

Malignant Lymphoma and Plasmacytoma 113

Leukemia 120

6   Pathological CSF Cell Findings in Cysts 129

V. Wieczorek, H. Kluge

References 133

Subject Index 135

1 Introduction

H. Kluge, V. Wieczorek, E. Linke, K. Zimmermann, O. W. Witte

In 1954, in Jena, in what was then the German Democratic Republic (GDR), J. Sayk of the Hans Berger Clinic for Psychiatry and Neurology developed the cell sedimentation chamber that was later named after him, working in collaboration with the Carl Zeiss company. This was followed by a worldwide surge in cytological study of cerebrospinal fluid (CSF) for diagnostic purposes. The Sayk method of obtaining cells from the CSF, in which cells are normally rare, by spontaneous sedimentation was the least traumatic technique that had been developed up to that time, and indeed remains so today. Cytological examination of the CSF became a routine method of clinical laboratory investigation with the application of the panoptic Pappenheim stain already in use for blood and bone marrow cells (a combination of the May-Grünwald eosin–methylene blue stain with the Giemsa azure II–eosin stain) to the cells obtained by Sayk's method.

By the early 1960s this technique, which originated in the Jena "school" of clinical CSF cytology of the late 1950s (J. Sayk, V. Wieczorek, R. M. Schmidt), was adopted by centers in Rostock (J. Sayk when he took up the chair there, R. Olischer, H. Meyer-Rienecker, later R. Lehmitz) and Halle (R. M. Schmidt after assuming the chair), while continuing to be practiced in Jena (V. Wieczorek, later H. Kluge). These three centers soon initiated a program of training and continuing education in CSF cytology for heads of clinical and research laboratories and for technical assistants in CSF laboratories throughout the GDR; the laboratories themselves joined together to form a "Working Group for the Diagnostic Study of the Cerebrospinal Fluid and Clinical Neurochemistry." The "Stadtroda Seminars in CSF Cytology," which provide training and continuing education in the field, were founded in 1984 on the initiative of E. Linke, then head of the laboratory in the Stadtroda Academic Hospital (Fachkrankenhaus), and have taken place annually since then with the collaboration and supervision of V. Wieczorek (Jena) and the support of K. Zimmermann (Arnsdorf-Dresden), H. Kluge (Jena), and H. Krause (Berlin).

The first nationwide German CSF symposium after the reunification of East and West Germany took place in Marburg in 1990 on the initiative of T. O. Kleine, E. Linke, and K. Zimmermann. In 1996, K. Felgenhauer, the Göttingen neurologist and President of the German Neurological Society, lent his support to the founding of the German Society for the Diagnostic Study of the Cerebrospinal Fluid and Clinical Neurochemistry, which is based in Jena. (We will refer to this Society by its German abbreviation, DGLN, which stands for *Deutsche Gesellschaft für Liquordiagnostik und Klinische Neurochemie e.V.*)

In 1987 and 1988, E. Linke and K. Zimmermann conducted round-robin CSF cytology tests in Stadtroda. In each test, 12 CSF specimens were examined by teams from 22 participating CSF laboratories from across the GDR. These were, to our knowledge, the first such tests to be conducted in Europe. From 1995 onward, Linke and Zimmermann were able to conduct tests of this type on a nationwide scale in Germany. These events, known as "On-Site Round-Robin Tests for Quality Assurance in CSF Diagnostic Studies" (*Ringversuche vor Ort zur Qualitätssicherung in der Liquordiagnostik*), have been held annually ever since with the collaboration of the DGLN and the support of INSTAND, Düsseldorf. They have already had a major, beneficial effect on the level of expertise in CSF cytology in Germany. Their most important benefit, however, has been the establishment of a *uniform standard of cell classification.*

Over the years, many participants in these seminars and round-robin tests in CSF cytology expressed a desire for an atlas of practical CSF cytology for the purposes of training and continuing medical education, which would be compiled from the extensive collection of cytological specimens assembled over a period of about 40 years by V. Wieczorek and H. Kluge. The authors have attempted to meet this desire by putting together the present text, in which the major emphasis is placed, as always, on the initial morphological study of cells in the CSF in a May–Grünwald–Giemsa preparation. This will presumably remain the preferred initial method of cytological study of the CSF for some time to come, as it is the essential prerequisite for all further cytological studies and thus must be done first as a selective diagnostic filter. The cell picture obtained by this classical method often yields important diagnostic information; even if it does not, it leads the way to specifically targeted further studies that will be beneficial for both diagnostic and scientific purposes.

Above all, this atlas is intended to provide an adequate grounding in CSF cytology for everyday practice in routine clinical laboratories and specialized CSF laboratories where such testing is done. The authors consider the need for such a text to be particularly pressing now that many of the previously independent CSF laboratories are being integrated into central laboratories whose technical and academic staff will need to be adequately trained in this subject. Chapters 2–6 will be especially useful for this purpose, because each of the numerous illustrations is accompanied by a brief discussion of the characteristic features and current World Health Organization (WHO) classification of the cell types depicted, and of the significance of the abnormal cytological findings in relation to the etiology and pathogenesis of the underlying disease.

We would like to point out that detailed descriptions of cytological methods have been omitted in this atlas, as these can be found without difficulty in the relevant literature, which is extensive. Furthermore, we feel obliged to explain that, in order to illustrate some of the less common types of CSF pleocytosis encountered in rarer diseases, we have had no choice but to display older specimens of slightly lesser quality. Up-to-date, advanced photographic techniques have been used to generate the illustrations in such cases and have greatly enhanced their appearance. For this, the authors are especially grateful to the staff of the Experimental Neurology Unit in the Hans Berger Clinics of Friedrich Schiller University, Jena, in particular to M. M. Kluska and C. Redecker, who expertly directed the photographic process using the clinical equipment of the Carl Zeiss company, Jena (Axioplan 2, AxioCam Hrc, AxioVision 3.1). We also thank Master Photographer W. Schumacher of Friedrich Schiller University for preparing the illustrations in timely fashion while the text was being written. Finally, we especially thank the technical staff of the CSF laboratory of the Jena Neurological Clinic for the preparation of the cytological specimens, in particular its long-serving Chief Technician, Ms. Adelheid Hoffmann.

Role of Practical (Classical) CSF Cytological Examination in the Overall Spectrum of CSF Diagnostic Studies

H. Kluge, V. Wieczorek, O. W. Witte, E. Linke, K. Zimmermann, E. Taub, S. Isenmann

Classical cytological examination based on the *Pappenheim stain (May–Grünwald–Giemsa stain)* remains the *centrally important first step* in the cytological evaluation of the CSF, because it generally enables at least an *initial categorization of the diagnosis* into one of the major types of neurological disease. In some cases, it even allows further *differential-diagnostic classification within a major disease category*, thereby yielding much more useful information than a simple "yes" or "no." However, classical cytological examination is rarely the final, conclusive test in differential diagnosis, because it usually fails to reveal the *specific disease* that is present, instead merely indicating the *class of diseases* to which it belongs. Yet this does not diminish its value as the point of departure from which the cytological diagnosis of the CSF will proceed. On the contrary, the information obtained by May–Grünwald–Giemsa staining is of crucial importance in determining whether other, more sensitive and more specific cytological marking techniques are *necessary* or *superfluous* for further evaluation. In many cases, decisions of this type can be made just on the basis of the clinical examination and the results of preliminary laboratory tests (e.g., findings in *other areas of the body* relevant to the patient's illness, and/or validated analysis of humoral markers in the blood and CSF).

In more concrete terms, classical CSF cytology is a rapid, inexpensive diagnostic technique that permits all of the following:

1. **Detection of infectious diseases of the central nervous system (CNS) and their classification into major categories.** Classical CSF cytological examination, when carried out either as an initial study or as a follow-up study in patients with CNS infections, yields information that determines which further test(s) should be done for identification of the pathogenic source (standard microbiological culture; enzyme-linked immunosorbent assay (ELISA) and blotting methods using pathogen-specific antibodies; molecular techniques, particularly hybridization/amplification with polymerase chain reaction (PCR), multiplex PCR, and blotting methods; immunocytochemical phenotyping of antibody-secreting cells, particularly with respect to immunoglobulin typing of activated B lymphocytes in the CSF).

2. **Demonstration of acute, or older, hemorrhages into the CSF spaces** that cannot be clearly revealed, or can no longer be clearly revealed, by neuroimaging studies (subarachnoid hemorrhage, hemorrhage accompanying inflammatory, traumatic, or neoplastic disease, etc.). Classical CSF cytological examination can also be used to distin-

guish true hemorrhage into the CSF space from the artifactual introduction of blood into the CSF.

3. **Detection of neoplastic cells and their (at least initial) classification by origin** in patients with an unknown or unclear oncological diagnosis (inadequate phenotyping of neoplastic cell populations of hematogenic origin, taken from the patient's blood, bone marrow, or lymph nodes; probable primary CNS lymphoma; unknown primary tumor; and unclear cases in which true neoplastic cells must be distinguished from lymphocytic activated forms, pre-neoplastic stages, non-neoplastic progenitor cells, and non-neoplastic stimulated cell forms). In such cases, classical CSF cytology can be followed by appropriate immunocytological phenotyping techniques for cell-line–specific proteins (characterization of cell lines by the expression or nonexpression of epithelial, oncofetal, neuroendocrine, mesenchymal, neuron-associated, and glia-associated antigens).

4. **Follow-up studies and treatment monitoring in patients** with pleocytosis and/or qualitative cellular changes in the CSF, as well as the monitoring of external ventricular drains for infection or inflammatory reaction to the catheter (material intolerance).

The remaining sections of this chapter, and the text sections introducing the illustrations in later chapters, contain more detailed information about the indications, utility, and limitations of the special tests mentioned in points 1–4, above, in addition to classical CSF cytological examination.

In addition, the cytological findings, together with the CSF cell count and protein concentration, may indicate the need for additional laboratory study of the noncellular components of the CSF (albumin quotient, intrathecal synthesis of various substances, humoral process markers, etc.). Cytological examination thus plays a key role in the *integrated* diagnostic evaluation of the CSF.

Over the past decade in particular, we have noticed a marked increase in the number of specimens of ventricular CSF obtained via *external ventricular drainage* by neurosurgeons in our referral area. The most important clinical consideration here is obligatory monitoring for *possible secondary catheter infections*, which can occur at any time, despite optimal hygienic precautions, because of colonization of the ventricular catheter with pathogenic organisms. Two further uses of ventricular CSF cytology are the *monitoring of reparative processes* and the detection of *incompatibility with the catheter material*. The cytological examination of ven-

tricular CSF with May–Grünwald–Giemsa staining is just as reliable as that of lumbar or cisternal CSF, because fluid obtained from all three of these areas has essentially the same cytological profile. The combination of cytological examination and standard microbiological culture of ventricular CSF constitutes an adequate battery of CSF tests when the purpose is to monitor for infection or for foreign-body reactions. The difference between the cytological picture of ventricular CSF and that of CSF from other sites is usually only quantitative: for certain structural and physiological reasons, surgical procedures and other disturbing factors in the ventricular system tend to produce a more marked *granulocytic pleocytosis* (neutrophilic and eosinophilic). This pleocytosis occurs in response to ventricular wall irritation, even in the absence of infection. In the authors' experience, the ventricular CSF cell count often exceeds 500 cells/μL, with more than 75 % neutrophilic granulocytes, even under broad-spectrum antibiotic coverage and in the absence of detectable microorganisms. In addition, macrophages of monocytic derivation are often found, as well as cells of epithelial/ependymal, mesenchymal, and endothelial origin and, occasionally, varieties of these cells that have been transformed into macrophages (cf. Chapter 4).

The fundamental observations that we have made in this section and in the remaining sections of this chapter, as well as in the introductory text preceding the illustrations of special cytological findings in the other chapters of this book, are based not only on our own experience but also on information that can be found in relevant chapters and literature cited in other specialized textbooks in the field. Some of these texts are fairly recent (Thomas 1998; Felgenhauer and Beuche 1999; Zettl *et al.* 2003, 2005), whereas others are older (Kölmel 1978; Dommasch and Mertens 1980; Schmidt 1987). Likewise, to complement our discussion of the cytological findings with the indispensable further information from other clinical neurosciences, we have made use of the basic literature in neuropathology (Cervos-Navarro and Ferszt 1989) and of the WHO classifications of tumors of the nervous system (Kleihues and Cavenee 2000; Radner *et al.* 2002). A number of cytological atlases of the CSF have been published, but none are recent: Oehmichen (1976), Kölmel (1978), Schmidt (1978), Den Hartog Jager (1980). A few of the major recent findings in basic science are mentioned in this book in the appropriate places. Finally, there is a list of older works at the end of the book, relating to the subject matter of Chapters 3–5, which were important milestones in the development of the Jena school of CSF cytology (Sayk *et al.*).

Diagnostic Use of Immunocytological Phenotyping Techniques in CSF Cytology

M. Wick, H. Kluge, E. Schulze, R. Lehmitz, M. M. Kluska

In the classical cytologic examination of the CSF, cell preparation with the May–Grünwald–Giemsa stain usually permits the basic identification and a fairly precise classification of malignant and inflammatory cell populations. Cells of these two types may be difficult to distinguish from one another, however, and subclassification is often not possible. Thus, the additional use of *immunocytological phenotyping techniques* may be necessary. When deciding whether to use such techniques, the CSF diagnostician must first ask *whether the potential findings will be helpful for diagnosis and treatment*, i.e., whether these techniques will really provide any clinical benefit. For example, if *myelogenous or lymphocytic neoplastic cell populations or immature preneoplastic stages* have already been detected in specimens of *blood, bone marrow, or lymph nodes*, so that the diagnosis of *myelogenous or lymphocytic leukemia or lymphoma* has already been made or ruled out, additional immunocytological phenotyping of the CSF cellular sediment is unnecessary. The same holds for *brain metastases* if the *primary tumor is already known.*

Thus, immunocytological phenotyping of CSF cells is indicated only for the *classification of atypical cells when a tumor of uncertain origin* or *primary CNS lymphoma* is suspected ("tumor-suspect" cells on May–Grünwald–Giemsa staining, particularly when only a few cells are seen), or for the *differentiation of lymphocytic-inflammatory from lymphocytic-neoplastic cell populations.*

Immunocytological phenotyping is recommended, although it is not indispensable, for the *quantification of subclasses of activated B lymphocytes* (B cells), particularly in *chronic inflammatory diseases*, if the May–Grünwald–Giemsa preparation reveals only a few activated lymphocytes, or only mildly stimulated ones. (For further details, see Chapter 3, Cytological Findings in Infectious and Inflammatory Diseases and the corresponding chapters in Zettl *et al.* 2003, 2005.)

The antibodies used for phenotyping are *the same for all techniques regardless of the tissue being studied, depending only on the particular cell lineage that is to be* demonstrated. They can be used for the study of CSF cells just as well as other tissues. A major *limiting factor* for the immunocytological phenotyping of CSF cells is the *amount of cellular sediment* that is available for study. This amount determines the *technique* that must be used. Each immunocytological marking requires 1000–10 000 "white cells," depending on the frequency of the specific cell population being sought; thus, *when the CSF contains only rare cells, flow cytometry is difficult or impossible to perform*, even with the use of double or triple antibody marking (see Diagnostic Use of Flow Cytometry in CSF Cytological Examination below). It can be done only if a large volume of CSF is centrifuged to increase the cellular concentration before cytometric testing.

Microscopic techniques for the phenotyping of *cellular sediment (immunofluorescence microscopy and immunocytochemical techniques)* require at least 1000 and preferably at least 5000 cells per marking. These techniques are carried out after cellular enrichment by sedimentation and provide usable results even when the CSF contains only rare, atypical cells of the type(s) to be demonstrated. However, multiple antibody marking is then difficult and, therefore, a larger number of sedimented specimens is required. (Our experience confirms this principle, especially in the case of "tumor-suspect" cells.)

If "tumor-suspect" and other atypical cells are seen in the May–Grünwald–Giemsa preparation and the CSF laboratory does not have the on-site capability for immunocytological phenotyping, or the necessary experience for it, we recommend that some of the excess CSF not needed for other tests be used to prepare more slides of air-dried, unstained sediment (the lower the total cell count, the more such slides should be made), and that these slides then be speedily sent to a specialized laboratory for phenotyping.

A comprehensive discussion of critical points concerning analytical evaluation, differential diagnostic clusters, and the corresponding antibody panels can be found in Thomas (1998) and Zettl *et al.* (2003, 2005).

Diagnostic Use of Flow Cytometry in CSF Cytology

E. Sindern, M. Wick, M. Roskos, M. Kiehntopf, H. Kluge

For the study of body fluids with a *high concentration of cells*, such as blood, flow cytometry is now well established as a routine diagnostic technique that has clear advantages over the traditional microscopic methods. Its potential application to the study of CSF is more limited, however, because normal CSF is *poor in cells*, with a white cell concentration generally no more than 1/1000 of that of blood. Whenever flow cytometric study of the CSF is both technically feasible and clinically indicated, it is recommended that it should be done in combination with a classical differential cytological examination of the CSF in a May–Grünwald–Giemsa preparation. The reasons for these general considerations are given below.

First, the flow cytometers now routinely used for hematology and urinalysis (ADVIA 120, CellDyn 3500 and 400, Sysmex UF-100) measure the cellular parameters of size, volume, surface area, granularity, and fluorescence with the use of two fluorescent dyes, phenanthridine for DNA and carbocyanin for cell membranes. They can be used to determine the total cell count of the CSF, as well as a differential cell count that includes erythrocytes (red blood cells [RBCs]), mononuclear cells (lymphocytes and monocytes), and polymorphonuclear cells (neutrophilic and eosinophilic granulocytes). The mononuclear cell count, however, includes only *normal* lymphocytes and monocytes. *Pathological* mononuclear cell populations, whose detection is often of crucial importance to neurological diagnosis, have extremely varied characteristics with respect to the analytical parameters measured by these cytometers. Activated lymphocytes (see Chapter 3), activated monocytes (including macrophages, see Chapter 4), many different types of tumor cell and tumor-suspect cell (including mitoses, see Chapter 5), bone marrow components, and epithelial cells (see Chapter 2) remain *undetected* by these cytometers, or else they are mistakenly assigned to one of the three categories mentioned. Therefore, no experienced CSF cytologist or responsible clinical neurologist can share the highly optimistic assessment of Aune *et al.* (2004), who consider a "CSF assay" with the ADVIA 120 apparatus to be an *acceptable alternative* to manual microscopic methods. One must rather agree with the more critical opinion of Strik *et al.* (2005), who consider the use of this apparatus acceptable only for emergency testing, and even then only in combination with a simultaneous cell preparation for microscopic analysis. As responsible clinical neurologists Strik et al. take a critical and objective view of the methodological and diagnostic limitations of flow cytometry.

Second, CSF flow cytometry coupled with *immunocytological* characterization of diagnostically relevant cell populations can certainly be of major diagnostic importance. In the remainder of this section, we will describe the technical principles and sphere of application of these techniques. The following conditions and details must be taken into consideration.

When the CSF specimen contains an *adequate number of cells for analysis* the clinical benefits of flow cytometry can be fully realized. Functionally distinct cell populations that are difficult or impossible to differentiate from one another with classical staining techniques can often be distinguished by flow cytometry based on varying amount of binding of fluorescence-marked monoclonal antibodies to their surface and intracellular antigens, because different cell populations bear antigens of different types and/or density (*immunological phenotyping*, cf. Diagnostic Use of Immunocytological Phenotyping Techniques in CSF Cytology). Furthermore, flow cytometry enables examination of *all* of the nucleated cells within the fluid volume being studied, and not just with a single antibody to a single antigen (a limitation of routinely used light microscopy) but with simultaneous *combinations of antibodies*, so-called "antibody panels," directed against two or three different antigens (*multiparametric analysis*). It provides a quantitative measure of the fluorescent activity of the labeled cells. The ability to examine a large number of cells at once enables detection of sparser cell populations than can be detected by microscopic techniques. Flow cytometry is a rapid, highly automated technique with steadily expanding uses for the examination of many different body fluids that contain cells. It has already been used for cell-kinetic and functional studies (enzyme activity, receptors, cell proliferation and cell cycles, inflammatory mediators, apoptosis, etc.).

However, flow cytometry, coupled with immunological characterization is difficult or impossible to carry out on CSF samples with *a normal or only mildly elevated* cell count. Each lumbar puncture yields an intrinsically limited quantity of CSF, lumbar punctures cannot be repeated *ad libitum*, and much of the CSF that is obtained must be sent for routine cytological, microbiological, and clinical chemical studies, so that, finally, little or none will remain for flow cytometry (a possible need for cell enrichment by centrifugation will only worsen the problem). These difficulties can sometimes be circumvented by sending only the acellular component of the centrifuged CSF for clinical chemistry; indeed, testing of this component for humoral markers even suffices to establish the diagnosis in some cases, obviating the need for flow cytometry. If enrichment by centrifugation is necessary to obtain enough cells for all of the antibody (or antibody panel) tests that are to be done, including negative controls, one must expect a loss of about 40% of the cells through the process of centrifugation—up to 30% of lymphocytes and granulocytes and up to 80% of monocytes. Furthermore, as flow cytometry involves the statistical sampling of cell populations, its results generally have a binomial distribution: this implies that, if only a few cells are available for analysis, the result will lie within a wide confidence interval, i.e., the information obtained by flow cytometry will be relatively imprecise. The coefficient of variation for the repeated analysis of a single cell population has been reported to be as high as 30% (depending on the population studied).

How many cells are needed for analysis with currently available equipment, and what are the current applications of flow cytometry in the examination of the CSF? In response to the first question, the number varies depending on the percentage of all CSF cells that is represented by the *particular cell population* to be studied, out of which at least 100–200 cells should be present to ensure a reliable analysis. This general principle allows a critical assessment of statements in the literature on threshold levels for the *total number of white cells*. According to Dux *et al.* (1994), the analysis of *lymphocyte subpopulations* with the FACS-II System requires at least 1000 CSF cells per antibody panel (account has already been taken of 30–40% cell loss through centrifugation). With a normal cell count of 1–5 cells/µL, this corresponds to a required CSF volume of approximately 2 mL for each antibody panel (including negative control). On the other hand, if a viral inflammatory process has elevated the CSF cell count to 200 cells/µL a 50 µL aliquot would already contain 10 000 cells and could be used for flow cytometry directly, without centrifugation. Sindern's laboratory, using the same apparatus, requires at least 2000 cells per antibody panel, including negative control. Kleine *et al.* (1994) report the ability to analyze eight lymphocytic subpopulations with a total of 3–5 mL of CSF in aliquots of 100 µL of native CSF, as long as the cell count exceeds 10/µL (yielding at least 1000 cells per aliquot). Wick (in Zettl *et al.* 2003, 2005) states that at least 10 000 cells are needed for immune phenotyping of rarer types of lymphocytes. The number of cells needed per antibody panel thus varies from 1000 to 10 000. If these cells are to be obtained from an aliquot of 50 µL of native CSF, then the CSF cell count must be at least 20/µL (at least 100/µL is desirable).

These quantitative requirements, the other disadvantages of flow cytometry mentioned above, and the fact that it can only be used to study a small number of cell populations per test limit the current clinical applicability of flow cytometry to the cytologic analysis of CSF. Indeed, CSF flow cytometry is routinely done in only a few clinical laboratories and is more commonly used as a research tool. It is usually used to study lymphocytic cell populations, as lymphocyte loss through centrifugation (up to 30%) is acceptably low and seems to affect all subpopulations equally. Studies of lymphocytic pleocytosis have revealed a compartmentalization of lymphocytic subpopulations between the blood and the CSF: the CSF contains a significantly higher percentage of CD3+ cells (T lymphocytes), CD4+ cells (helper T lymphocytes), and CD4+CD29+ cells (activated helper-memory T lymphocytes) than the blood, which, in turn, contains a higher percentage of CD19+ cells (B lymphocytes), CD8+ cells (suppressor T lymphocytes), and CD4+CD45RA+ cells (naïve helper T lymphocytes). These differences are *independent* of the underlying condition. CSF of patients with relapsing-remitting multiple sclerosis (MS) has been found to contain a significantly higher percentage of CD19+ and CD4+CD29+ cells than that of patients with viral meningitis, viral encephalitis, or other, noninflammatory diseases of the nervous system. Most CD3+ cells in the CSF express the chemokine receptor CXCR3; in patients with MS, the degree of CXCR3 expression correlates with the extent of active inflammation revealed by magnetic resonance imaging (MRI) and perhaps reflects preferential recruitment of activated cells from the blood into the CSF (Oreja-Guevara *et al.* 1998, Sindern *et al.* 2002, Sindern 2004).

These findings, however, cannot yet be put to clinical use, nor does our current knowledge of the different lymphocytic composition of the CSF in various neurological diseases (mostly infectious/inflammatory) have any immediate clinical relevance beyond its usefulness in answering specific scientific questions. There is a potential future clinical application for CSF flow cytometry in the differential diagnosis of neoplastic meningitis.

Further information on CSF flow cytometry can be found in the relevant chapters in the cited literature (Thomas 1998, Zettl *et al.* 2003, 2005)

Proper Handling of CSF Specimens Before Cytological Examination

H. Kluge, M. Roskos, E. Linke, V. Wieczorek, E. Taub, S. Isenmann

The importance of proper handling of CSF specimens before cytological examination is easily understood as soon as one grasps the single most important reason for cell damage after lumbar puncture. The CSF normally contains little protein and only a few cells and thus mostly *lacks* the two main pH buffer systems that are present in blood, namely *cell surfaces and a high protein concentration*. Practically the *sole buffering capacity of the CSF* is derived from the *bicarbonate/carbon dioxide system*. A drop of CSF suspended from the lumbar puncture needle *gives up* its carbon dioxide content to the surrounding air because of the *steep partial pressure gradient for carbon dioxide* and thereby spontaneously *loses* the only pH buffering capacity that it has. Within seconds, therefore, the pH rises from 7.32–7.36 (normal CSF range) to alkaline values of 7.8 and higher. If the CSF is not very bloody (as in most normal and pathological specimens) and the CSF protein concentration is below 3000 mg/L, then, regardless of the white cell count, the elevated pH in combination with *active catabolic mechanisms* will cause a *considerable degree of cell damage and cell loss* even at this early stage. (The old aphorism about the CSF being a "hostile environment for cells" is misleading, as this is true only of CSF exposed to air.) On the other hand, bloody CSF with a high protein content contains adequate buffers, i.e., pH-stabilizing ampholytes on erythrocyte surfaces and protein molecules, so that the pH does not rise as rapidly and cell damage does not occur till much later. Experienced cytologists are well acquainted with this phenomenon and can obtain a diagnostically useful preparation and differential cell count from a bloody specimen as long as 4–6 hours after lumbar puncture. After a longer interval this is no longer possible because of cell loss and artifact formation.

The *method of cell sedimentation* is another *important factor affecting cell stability* (for details see below). Spontaneous sedimentation, e.g., in the Sayk chamber, is less damaging than cellular centrifugation, whose harmful effect is increased if the cells have already been damaged previously by medical treatment or by having been left standing too long after the lumbar puncture. The strict observance of a time limit (see below) is thus all the more important nowadays, when cell sedimentation is almost always done with a cell centrifuge. The *storage temperature of CSF* should be *between 5 °C and 12 °C* to minimize cell damage. Lower temperatures may lead to cold lysis, whereas higher temperatures accelerate the catabolic mechanisms mentioned above.

The best *receptacles and transport containers for CSF* are sterile, sealed *polypropylene test tubes*. Polycarbonate test tubes adsorb various substances to their surface, e.g., IgG, whereas glass test tubes should not be used because they adsorb cells and therefore artifactually alter the cell count. EDTA and sodium fluoride test tubes also impair cytological examination.

Keeping to a time limit from the moment of the lumbar puncture until the cytological examination is important not only because of progressive cell damage, but also because any cells present (particularly in CSF pleocytosis) can damage, or bind to, sensitive noncellular substances used as *diagnostic markers*, thereby preventing their detection. Aliquots of CSF that are to be used for diagnostic marker studies should have all cells removed as soon as the CSF specimen arrives in the laboratory. Taking into account all of the mechanisms that can damage cells, it can be concluded that the cytological examination of the CSF should take place no later than 2 hours after lumbar puncture. Experienced CSF cytologists can provide useful diagnostic information even after a time interval of 3 hours, but at 4 hours any findings must be accompanied by statement of caution.

For all these reasons, *central* cytological laboratories that process specimens from a wide referral area (and, of course, central laboratories that perform cytologic examination along with other tests) must establish a strict set of rules for specimen handling, both externally (at the referring hospital and in the transport system) and within the laboratory (assignment of specimens for processing, maintenance of technical standards). These rules should be adapted to local conditions. Referring physicians, in particular, must realize that lumbar punctures cannot be repeated at will, especially because of patient discomfort and the likelihood of postpuncture reactions, and therefore specimens must be carefully handled from the moment of lumbar puncture until they arrive in the laboratory.

There are other considerations that the physician should be aware of when taking specimens of ventricular CSF from external drainage systems. The (approximately) 2 mL of CSF lying between the catheter tip and the point of removal of specimens may have undergone secondary changes, as this portion of fluid has been lying outside the ventricular system for some time (the length of time depends on the volume of drainage per hour as well as on the diameter and length of the drainage tubing). This should be removed and discarded if possible. Other recommendations for the removal of ventricular CSF specimens can be found in the relevant chapters in Zettl *et al.* (2003, 2005).

The basic cytological examination (cell count, differential cell picture, and total protein) requires *a minimum of 2 mL of CSF*, though the precise amount may vary between laboratories. More CSF is needed if the suspected diagnosis calls for further specialized cytological testing (immunocytochemistry or flow cytometry). In such cases, the referring physician should contact the CSF laboratory for advice *before carrying out the lumbar puncture*. The same holds if tests are to be performed on solutes both in the acellular component of CSF and in the autologous serum (quotients of albumin, immunoglobulins, etc.). Our daily experience shows it is essential for CSF laboratories to provide *detailed information* to all referring institutions (departments of neurology, neurosurgery, anesthesiology, pediatrics, and psychiatry; medical oncology wards; etc.) about the proper handling of specimens and the required minimum volumes of CSF and autologous serum (if the serum is to be tested).

Cell Preparation (Sedimentation) and Staining

H. Kluge, M. Roskos, M. M. Kluska

The preparation of the cell sediment is among the more difficult technical components of the cell enrichment process because it is subject to a number of potential disturbances. *The Sayk method of spontaneous cell sedimentation*, which is mainly used to obtain populations of easily damaged, highly activated large-sized cells, is today still the best method for the *preservation of cellular structure*, superior in this respect to all methods involving filtration or centrifugation. The literature contains many quantitative and qualitative comparisons of these methods; here it will suffice to mention the representative and comprehensive paper by Lehmitz and Kleine (1994).

Nonetheless, improvements in *centrifugation techniques* over the years have made some of these techniques nearly as good at preserving cell structure as spontaneous sedimentation, with the further advantages of rapidity and constancy of technical parameters. Standardized centrifugation techniques are now in wide use; the most popular cell centrifuges are those manufactured by *Shandon Labortechnik* (Frankfurt, Germany) and *Hettich* (Tuttlingen, Germany).

Among the cell preparations shown in this cytological atlas, those produced before 1990 (the majority) were all made with Sayk's method of spontaneous cell sedimentation. From 1990 until about 1993, the authors made parallel preparations with the Sayk method and with cell centrifugation techniques, in an effort to raise the quality of the latter to the standard set by the former by modifying the centrifugation parameters and adding certain cell-protective substances. In these trials, we were indeed able to produce centrifuged cell preparations of acceptably similar quality to those made with the Sayk method. Yet we must stress that the centrifugation technique used by us and described further below, like any other centrifugation technique, cannot be applied in rote, unvarying fashion to every single specimen; rather, it must be optimally adapted to each specimen to obtain the best result. This is particularly true when an initial preparation has already been made and turns out to be of poor quality. The technical parameters that we give here for our "Jena version" of the technique should therefore be understood as rough guidelines derived from experience, allowing room for flexible application.

The particular variant of the cell centrifugation technique that we developed employs the *UNIVERSAL 32 cell centrifuge* with an angle chamber system (manufactured by *Hettich*, Tuttlingen, Germany) and is based on *one-step centrifugation* without any preliminary centrifugation enrichment of the type previously used for CSF specimens with a low cell count (two-step centrifugation). If the specimens have been handled properly before analysis (proper transport, keeping to time limits, etc., see above), this one-step technique yields diagnostically useful results without the cell loss and possible cell deformation caused by preliminary centrifugation. The technical details are as follows:

1. Centrifugation parameters for cell sedimentation and CSF volumes to be used

Among the centrifugation programs that we tested, the following were found to produce an *acceptably low* amount of cell damage:

100 × g (930 rpm with the above-mentioned centrifuge) for 3 minutes

or 50 × g (660 rpm) for 4 minutes.

The former is recommended for routine use. The cell yield for CSF specimens *with cell counts under 3/μL* was 25–35 %. Our deliberate use of a relatively low centrifugal acceleration to avoid cell damage explains why this cell yield is lower than that obtained by Lehmitz and Kleine (1994) in a two-step process using vertical cell chambers and an acceleration of 250 × g for 3 minutes.

We generally used a standardized *final fluid volume of 450 μL per angle chamber*. Out of this volume,

400 µL consisted of CSF and a variable amount of diluent depending on the cell count; the remaining 50 µL consisted of the required additives described below. A simple calculation shows that 400 µL of CSF with a cell count of 2/µL and a 25% cell yield will provide 200 cells, an adequate number for cytologic analysis. If there are fewer than 2 cells/µL, a higher CSF volume of up to 800 µL can be used, as this amount of fluid can still be taken up by the filter card. If the cell count is higher than 2/µL, a smaller quantity of CSF is used, together with the additives mentioned below for a final volume of 400 µL.

2. Accessories, additives, and staining

The procedure outlined above utilizes *angle chambers of 8.7 mm diameter (sedimentation surface area 60 mm^2)*, the corresponding *filter cards*, and *Polysine-coated object carriers* (for the May–Grünwald–Giemsa stain) or *Super Frost Color object carriers* (for immunocytochemical stains).

Protein additives are needed for pH buffering and cell stabilization if the *CSF cell count is below 10/µL* and its *protein content is below 3000 mg/L* (see Proper Handling of CSF Specimens Before Cytological Examination). The protein concentration can always be raised well above 3000 mg/L, if necessary, by adding *50 µL* of freshly obtained and re-centrifuged *normal serum* (which is readily available in all laboratories and contains about 70 g/L of total protein) to the 400-µL specimen. (There is no need to use autologous serum.) The protein concentration of a specimen treated in this way will be approximately 7800 mg/L plus the protein concentration of the original CSF specimen. Antibiotics and protein-rich culture media were used at one time as additives to CSF for centrifugation, but these substances are both expensive and of no benefit at all, as the cytological preparation must be accomplished rapidly in any case if it is to be diagnostically useful. *Bloody CSF with many cells* should be diluted by mixing an aliquot of CSF of the appropriate size with a 10:1 mixture of normal saline and serum.

The air-dried preparation is then stained in standard fashion for CSF sediment, with *May-Grünwald solution for 2–3 minutes*, then with *Giemsa solution for 10–15 minutes*. These times should be taken as guidelines and not as dogma.

The CSF Cytology Report: Consensus Reporting Form of the German Society for the Diagnostic Study of the Cerebrospinal Fluid and Clinical Neurochemistry for Use in On-Site Round-Robin Tests

E. Linke, H. Kluge

The creation of a standardized reporting form for CSF cytology was discussed in 1991 at the founding meeting of the (German) Working Group for the Diagnostic Study of the Cerebrospinal Fluid and Clinical Neurochemistry. The chief participants were neurologists and heads of CSF laboratories who were all well acquainted with the diagnostic importance of CSF cytology in clinical practice and who had themselves published important work in this area (Sayk, Wieczorek, Olischer; Schmidt and Kölmel; authors of earlier cytologic atlases of the CSF; and others). The Working Group produced a consensus reporting form, which is reproduced in English in Figure 1.**1**.

The consensus reporting form has been used since 1995 in the nationwide on-site round-robin tests that first began in the Stadtroda CSF laboratory (E. Linke and K. Zimmermann, cf. Role of Practical (Classical) CSF Cytological Examination and the chapter devoted to this subject in Zettl *et al.* 2003, 2005). Figure 1.**1** shows the current version, which can be used to record not only the cytological findings (cell populations present and absent) but also the evaluating cytolo-gist's judgment of the findings of the previous examiner.

All participants agreed at the outset that the form should have spaces to indicate the presence or absence of *monocytes, activated monocytes, phage and granulocyte subpopulations, and lymphocytes.* There was considerable discussion, however, about the many subtypes of *lymphoid cells* that are seen in May–Grünwald–Giemsa preparations, and their many transitional forms, which are nearly impossible to classify precisely and reproducibly. The presence of these immunocompetent subpopulations in the CSF is indeed evidence of an inflammatory reaction, but it does not imply anything else about the differential diagnostic classification; therefore, it was finally agreed that all these cell types would be designated by the collective term "activated lymphocytes," which is meant to encompass all *transformed, non-neoplastic lymphocytic cell types.* A distinct category was maintained only for *plasma cells*, which can be considered the last transformational stage of the lymphocytic series—even though subtypes of plasma cells, too, are sometimes difficult to distinguish from activated lymphocytes in classical cytological preparations. The latter problem is discussed in greater detail in Chapter 3. The *differential diagnostic classification* of lymphocytic subpopulations is possible only with immunocytochemical techniques, as discussed above and in the relevant chapters of Zettl *et al.* (2003, 2005).

The participants also had varying ideas about the classification of neoplastic cell populations. It was finally agreed that there would be a space to indicate the presence or absence of *neoplastic and tumor-suspect cells*, as well as separate blank lines where the examiner could further specify the type of malignant cell in cases of suspected *lymphoma* or *leukemia*, if desired. The extensive presentation of neoplastic cell popula-

tions in Chapter 5 of this book contains the type of information that is to be specified on these lines in relevant cases.

The term *surface epithelium*, discussed further in Chapter 2 (see Cells and Cell Clusters From the Structures Enclosing the CSF Space), refers to the cells and cellular networks that form the boundaries of the CSF space (subarachnoid space). The need to include *bone marrow cells* on the reporting form is justified in Chapter 2 (see Lumbar Puncture Artifacts). An indication of the possible presence of *erythrocytes*, due to a real or artifactual admixture of blood, is clearly indispensable as well. Finally, the last line is reserved for mention of *other cell types*, if present.

Institut für Standardisierung und Dokumentation
im medizinischen Laboratorium e.V.
INSTAND
Düsseldorf, Germany

On-Site Round-Robin Tests in CSF Cytology

EVALUATION FORM

Name of Participant: Microscope / Workbench No.::

	Slide 1		Slide 2		Slide 3		Slide 4		
	qualitative		qualitative		qualitative		qualitative		
	Previous finding	Your finding	Previous finding	Your finding	Previous finding	Your finding	Previous finding	Your finding	
Monocytes	□	○	□	○	□	○	□	○	*Slide 1* Cytological diagnosis:
Activated monocytes	□	○	□	○	□	○	□	○	Evaluation*:
Leukophages	□	○	□	○	□	○	□	○	Differentiation: Verbal:
Lipophages	□	○	□	○	□	○	□	○	Remarks:
Erythrophages	□	○	□	○	□	○	□	○	
Hemosiderophages	□	○	□	○	□	○	□	○	*Slide 2* Cytological diagnosis:
Bacteriophages/bacteria	□	○	□	○	□	○	□	○	Evaluation*:
Neutrophilic granulocytes	□	○	□	○	□	○	□	○	Differentiation: Verbal:
Eosinophilic granulocytes	□	○	□	○	□	○	□	○	Remarks:
Lymphocytes	□	○	□	○	□	○	□	○	*Slide 3* Cytological diagnosis:
Activated lymphocytes (= all transformed lymphocytic non-neoplastic cell types, e.g., lymphoid cells with darkly staining cytoplasm)	□	○	□	○	□	○	□	○	Evaluation*:
Plasma cells	□	○	□	○	□	○	□	○	Differentiation: Verbal:
Tumor and tumor-suspect cells	□	○	□	○	□	○	□	○	Remarks:
	□	○	□	○	□	○	□	○	
Surface epithelium	□	○	□	○	□	○	□	○	*Slide 4* Cytological diagnosis:
Bone marrow cells	□	○	□	○	□	○	□	○	Evaluation*:
Erythrocytes	□	○	□	○	□	○	□	○	Differentiation: Verbal:
Other cell types	□	○	□	○	□	○	□	○	Remarks:
									Signatures:

* Evaluations: 1: Differentiation or assessment correct
2: Differentiation or assessment basically correct but in need of minor corrections
3: Differentiation incorrect   3a: important cell population not recognized
3b: cell population designated as present when in fact absent

Fig. 1.1 On-site Round-Robin Tests in CSF Cytology:–Evaluation Form

2 Cell Populations in the Normal Cerebrospinal Fluid

H. Kluge, E. Linke, V. Wieczorek, K. Zimmermann, H.-J. Kuehn

The *normal lumbar cerebrospinal fluid* (CSF) obtained by an *uncomplicated lumbar puncture* has a cell count of up to 5/µL, consisting exclusively of *lymphocytes* and *monocytes* in a ratio of approximately 70:30 (in sediment obtained by centrifugation) or 60:40 (after spontaneous sedimentation in a Sayk chamber, cf. Lymphocytes and Monocytes below). Rarely, normal CSF obtained in this way will contain cells or cell clusters belonging to the structures that enclose the CSF space. These cells, designated as *surface epithelium* in the consensus reporting form in Figure 1.**1** (see also The CSF Cytology Report, Chapter 1 and Cells and Cell Clusters from the Structures Enclosing the CSF Space below),

are more commonly seen after *complicated lumbar punctures* and in *ventricular CSF*. Their presence in lumbar CSF is to be considered a secondary effect of manipulation, i.e., as a **CSF artifact**. Further artifactual findings include *bone marrow cells* obtained by unintended aspiration of the marrow space as well as *skin and cartilage cells* (see Lumbar Puncture Artifacts below).

Possible secondary artifacts due to contamination of the specimen after lumbar puncture (bacteria, fungi, dust particles, etc.) are not discussed in this chapter. The possibly artifactual admixture of blood in the CSF is discussed in Chapter 4.

Lymphocytes and Monocytes

The *lymphocytes* in the cellular sediment of *normal* CSF stained with the May–Grünwald–Giemsa method are nonactivated, small isomorphic cells with a diameter of 5–8 µm. The round or mildly oval, turbid or coarsely granulated nucleus is surrounded by a very thin rim of cytoplasm, which is either practically indiscernible (such lymphocytes are said to have "naked nuclei") or just wide enough to be visible. The cytoplasm is clear or, at most, mildly basophilic (Fig. 2.**1**).

Immunocytochemical methods of cell differentiation (flow cytometry) reveal that about 93 % of lymphocytes in normal CSF are *T lymphocytes* and about 1 % are *B lymphocytes*. The distinction between these two types of cell is important in the differential diagnosis of inflammatory and infectious diseases. Venous blood, in contrast, contains 60–80 % T lymphocytes and 10–30 % B lymphocytes.

Activated lymphocytes (activated B lymphocytes; many earlier authors classified these cells according to their cytoplasmic size and basophilia as a highly heterogeneous category of *lymphoid cells*, see Chapter 3, Cytological Findings in Infectious and Inflammatory Diseases) are rarely present in normal CSF, and their final differentiated type—the *plasma cell*—is never found in it. These cell types and the question of the origin of normal and activated lymphocytes in CSF are discussed in Chapter 3.

The *monocytes* in the cellular sediment of *normal* CSF stained with the May–Grünwald–Giemsa method are of *hematogenic (monocytopoietic) origin*. Before passing into the CSF, however, they are present as "free" cells in the extracellular spaces of the meninges (including the stroma of the choroid plexus). Here, under pathological conditions, they may become transformed into activated monocytes and then into macrophages (see Chapter 4). As these monocytes are surrounded by a quite different milieu than blood, and because they have to migrate twice to find their way into the CSF (first across the vascular endothelium and then through the epithelial/ependymal cell layers), "normal" CSF monocytes have a highly varied morphology; at times, they almost resemble activated monocytes. With diameters of 15–20 µm, they are about four times as large as the normal CSF lymphocytes. The peripherally located nucleus is oval, or kidney- or horseshoe-shaped, or lobulated, and sometimes contains pale nucleoli. The cytoplasm is smoky gray or, at most, mildly basophilic near the cell membrane. Any basophilic coloring of the cytoplasm, or the occasional appearance of a few vesicular structures within it, indicates an incipient activated state. Figure 2.**2** shows diverse structural variants of "normal" CSF monocytes surrounding five normal lymphocytes in the center of the figure.

Although this chapter is principally devoted to *normal* cell morphology, we have included some normal forms and contrasting *activated forms* of lymphocytes and monocytes in Figure 2.**3** for didactic purposes. Note the differences between normal and activated types with respect to cell size and shape, nuclear size and shape, and above all, cytoplasmic structure and staining. Activated monocytes are sometimes considerably larger than the ones shown in Figure 2.**3** (see the cytological illustrations in Chapters 3 and 4 for examples).

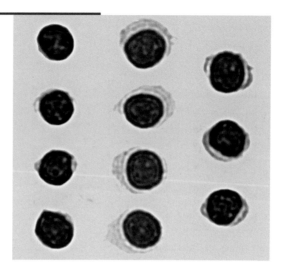

Fig. 2.**1** Nonactivated lymphocytes in normal CSF. Left column: lymphocytes with "naked nuclei," i.e., the cytoplasm is barely discernible as a clear or only slightly colored rim around the nucleus. Middle column: lymphocytes with a significantly larger amount of clear cytoplasm. Right column: lymphocytes with a thin, mildly basophilic rim of cytoplasm (incipient activation).

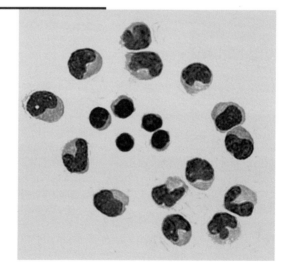

Fig. 2.**2** Nonactivated monocytes in normal CSF (outer circle of cells), some of which show early signs of activation, and, for comparison, lymphocytes with a thin, mildly basophilic rim of cytoplasm (the five cells in the center).

Fig. 2.**3** An illustration of different cell types to demonstrate the cytological differences between nonactivated and activated lymphocytes and monocytes in the CSF. First column from left: nonactivated or only mildly activated monocytes. Second column from left: monocytes in various stages of activation. First column from right: nonactivated or only mildly activated lymphocytes. Second column from right: activated lymphocytes, some of which are undergoing transformation to plasma cells (see Chapter 3, Cytological Findings in Infectious and Inflammatory Disease).

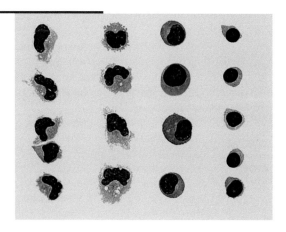

Cells and Cell Clusters From the Structures Enclosing the CSF Space

The cells described in this section, which are designated as "*surface epithelium*" in the consensus reporting form in Figure 1.**1**, mainly consist of *plexus epithelial cells, ependymal* and *endothelial cells,* and *meningeal cells of mesenchymal origin* (meningeal connective tissue cells). They can be found in normal CSF as an artifact of lumbar puncture, in CSF of hydrocephalic children, and in CSF altered by certain pathological conditions (e.g., infectious or other processes affecting the structures that enclose the CSF space).

When present as an *artifact of lumbar puncture,* cells of these types are derived from the injured meningeal layers and/or the other tissues along the trajectory of the lumbar puncture needle. If they are recognized as an artifact, they are to be interpreted as a normal finding. Epithelial and ependymal cells are more commonly seen in such cases than the other two cell types mentioned above. Cells of all four types can display the morphological features of their cell population of origin when seen on cytological examination of the CSF, as long as the time interval between the lumbar puncture and the cytological preparation is not prolonged (see Chapter 1, Proper Handling of CSF Specimens Before Cytological Examination).

Epithelial cells are often seen in large clusters. The chromatin-rich nucleus is mostly isomorphic, round to lightly oval, and mainly peripherally located. The cytoplasm is acidophilic. The more fragile *ependymal cells* have similar-looking nuclei, which, however, are more often pyknotic in shape, and a paler cytoplasm, often with peripheral fraying. *Endothelial cells* are more elongated and usually have an oblong, oval nucleus. *Cells of mesenchymal origin* from the connective tissue of the meningeal layers often display a fibrillary structure in their predominantly acidophilic cytoplasm.

Regardless of the length of the interval between the lumbar puncture and further processing of the CSF specimen, the local environment of these cells is altered when they are separated from their tissues of origin and set free in the CSF. They may thus undergo secondary changes that make them barely recognizable. An excessively long interval between the lumbar puncture and further processing will, of course, lead to yet more cell degeneration. As these complicating phenomena make these four cell types difficult to tell apart from each other, and because their presence in CSF is merely an artifact and thus of no diagnostic significance, CSF cytologists are agreed that they can be grouped together under the collective heading *surface epithelium.* The final (descriptive, not merely numerical) cytology report should always state explicitly that the presence of these cells is an artifact, to distinguish this situation from the rarer finding of *activated or transformed cells* of these four types, which may possess *diagnostic significance* (see Chapter 4). This will occur mainly under *pathological conditions* associated with *disease-induced destruction of meningeal and parenchymal tissue* (trauma, subarachnoid hemorrhage, cerebral infarction, infection/inflammation, and hydro-cephalus induced by any of these processes).

These cells are also more often found in *ventricular CSF samples,* because of the greater degree of manipulation required to obtain the specimen. The four types of surface epithelial cells are subject to marked morphological and functional alteration when their presence in the CSF is due to disease-induced tissue destruction. The reason for this is that these cell populations, which already possess a certain degree of functional differentiation owing to their location, become further *differentiated (transformed)* in the setting of additional, disease-induced changes in their local environment. Surface epithelial cells, if present in the CSF, may thus be capable of phagocytosis (i.e., they may have become transformed into *macrophages*). The disease-induced changes in the local environment generally cause a massive quantitative and qualitative increase of transformation-promoting factors in the CSF space. The processes by which cells are transformed into macrophages and the difficulties encountered by the CSF cytologist in interpreting the resulting cell pictures are discussed in Chapter 4.

Figures 2.**4**–2.**9** show surface epithelial cells as they are found in lumbar CSF, usually as a puncture artifact, and in ventricular CSF. Signs of cell activation are indicated, including the separation of individual cells from cell clusters, increased polychromasia, and hyperchromasia in the cytoplasm.

Fig. 2.**4** A cluster of plexus epithelial cells with acidophilic cytoplasm, which is mildly basophilic and partly vacuolated at the periphery (secretion?), and an isomorphic, rounded, chromatin-rich nucleus.

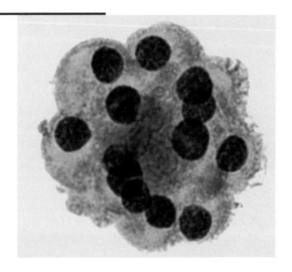

Fig. 2.**5** Clusters of plexus cells affected by mild degenerative changes. The cytoplasm is fragmented and contains acidophilic granules; the nuclei show incipient deformation and disintegration.

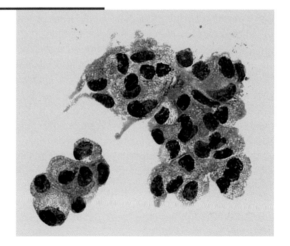

Fig. 2.**6** Epithelial cluster of isomorphic chromaffin cells with incipient cell separation at the edges. A monocyte and a few degenerated granulocytes are seen in the vicinity (remission phase of meningitis).

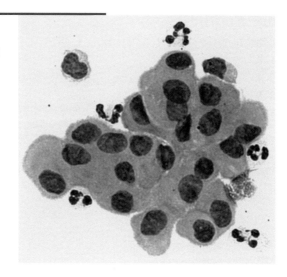

Fig.2.**7** Ependymal clusters and free individual cells, possibly incipient activation to phagocytic cell types (see Chapter 4).

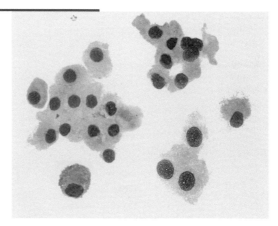

Fig. 2.**8** Cluster and doublet of isomorphic, hyperchromatic, activated cells of mesenchymal or ependymal origin in a patient with subarachnoid hemorrhage. A tendency toward separation of individual cells can be seen in the cluster; differentiation to erythrophages is likely (see Chapter 4).

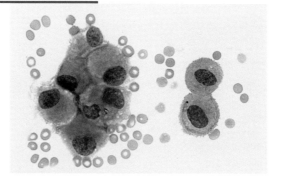

Fig. 2.**9** Ependymal or mesenchymal cluster in acute subarachnoid hemorrhage containing activated acidophilic, reticulated cytoplasmic structures that contain vesicles. There is incipient cell separation with probable transformation to macrophages (see Chapter 4).

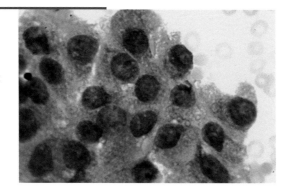

Lumbar Puncture Artifacts:
Bone Marrow Components, Cartilage Cells, etc.

If the patient's spine is anatomically abnormal or is injured, or if the patient's posture during the lumbar puncture is insufficiently relaxed, there is a greater likelihood that the lumbar puncture needle will strike against bone and that *bone marrow components* will be aspirated together with the CSF. Other cell types and tissues that may appear in the CSF as an artifact of lumbar puncture are *cartilage cells, skin cells, capillaries* and *subdermal connective tissue cells.* Capillaries of the plexus choroideus or of ventricle walls are occasionally seen in ventricular CSF.

Among the unintentionally aspirated *bone marrow cells,* the CSF cytologist may find the many different immature forms associated with *erythropoiesis* (ranging from proerythroblasts to normoblasts), *myelo-*

poiesis (from myeloblasts to metamyelocytes), *mono-cytopoiesis* (from monoblasts to promonocytes), and *thrombocytopoiesis* (from megakaryoblasts to megakaryocytes). If these cell types are not recognized, they can easily be *misdiagnosed,* e.g., as neoplastic or tumor-suspect cells (cf. the tumor cell criteria in Chapter 5).

Examples of these immature forms are shown in Figures 2.**10**–2.**15**. Immature progenitor stages in the lymphocytic series are shown in Figure 2.**16** and in some of the illustrations in other parts of this book dealing with infectious and inflammatory processes (see Chapter 3) and leukemic meningitis (Chapter 5, Leukemia). Typical cartilage cells are shown in Figure 2.**17**, and capillaries in ventricular CSF are shown in Figure 2.**18**.

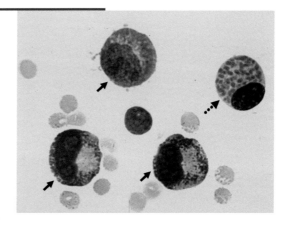

Fig. 2.**10** Promyelocytes in various stages of maturation (solid arrows) and an immature eosinophilic myelocyte (broken arrow).

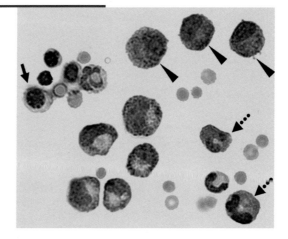

Fig. 2.**11** Normoblast (solid arrow); myeloblasts (arrowheads); left, promyelocytes and eosinophil precursors; below right, two eosinophilic granulocytes (broken arrows) and a neutrophilic granulocyte with a band-shaped nucleus.

Fig. 2.**12** Erythroblast (broken arrow); metamyelocyte (arrowhead); promyelocytes (solid arrows).

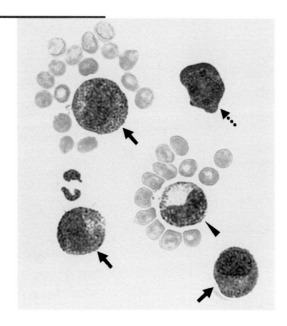

Fig. 2.**13** Myelocyte and, below, a possible megakaryoblast (megakaryocyte?).

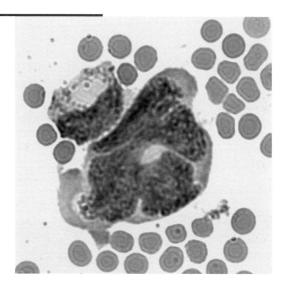

Fig. 2.**14** Bone marrow components in the CSF as an artifact of lumbar puncture. Various precursor stages of hematopoiesis are seen: promyelocytes in different stages of maturation; polychromatic normoblasts (single cells and two nests of cells); orthochromatic normoblasts as individual cells and nests of cells.

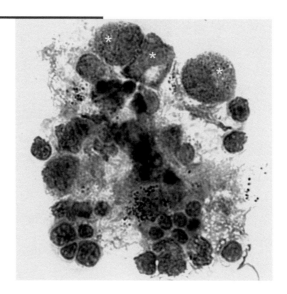

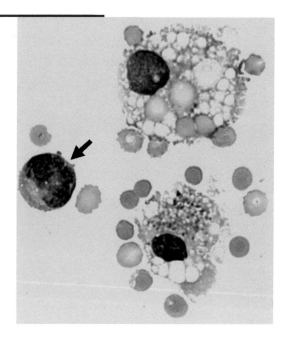

Fig. 2.**15** Progenitor cell (arrow), possibly of the monocytic (hematogenous phagocytic) lineage, in a patient with subarachnoid hemorrhage past the acute stage. There are also two erythro-hemosiderophages containing considerable amounts of lipid (other bone marrow cells were found in the remainder of the cytological preparation).

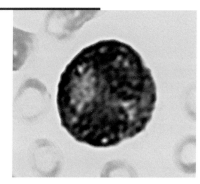

Fig. 2.**16** Progenitor stage of a plasma cell in amitotic division. This cytological preparation also contained other bone marrow cells.

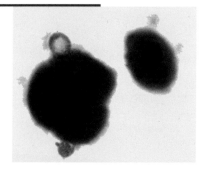

Fig. 2.**17** Cartilage cells, single and in a cluster: coarsely structured, round to oval nucleus, large and deeply stained cytoplasmic areas with color alternating between blue and red. For size, compare with the neighboring erythrocytes.

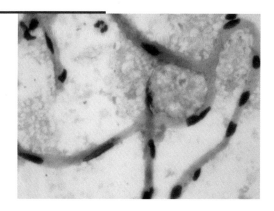

Fig. 2.**18** Capillaries (from the choroid plexus or the ventricle walls) in ventricular CSF obtained through an external drain after a neurosurgical procedure. Elongated endothelial cells with a typical oval nucleus are seen.

3 Pathological CSF Cell Findings in Infectious and Inflammatory Diseases of the Central Nervous System

V. Wieczorek, H. Kluge, E. Linke, R. Lehmitz, M. Gajda, H. Guhlmann, S. Isenmann

The cellular response in the CSF provides the neurologist with important diagnostic clues to infectious and (less commonly) noninfectious inflammatory diseases of the nervous system, such as meningitis, meningo-encephalitis, encephalomyelitis, and abscesses, as well as to diseases that are primarily neither infectious nor inflammatory, yet trigger a secondary inflammatory reaction (e.g., reactive pleocytosis due to subarachnoid hemorrhage, traumatic brain injury, highly malignant central nervous system [CNS] tumors). Cytological examination of the CSF in these pathological conditions reveals granulocytes, lymphocytes and their various activated forms, and monocytes and their activated forms. These cell populations are described in detail in Chapter 2 (Lymphocytes and Monocytes), the first section of this chapter (Granulocytes and Activated Forms of the Lymphocytic Series), and in Chapter 4.

The total CSF cell count and the qualitative and quantitative composition of the cells enable the CSF cytologist to assess the temporal course of the cellular response to the inflammatory stimulus. This kind of information *rarely if ever suffices for an exact diagnosis*, but the constellation of findings will often be *characteristic of a particular variety of disease course and a particular class of pathogen* and thus point the way to further, more *specific testing* for viral and bacterial *pathogens* and for cellular and humoral *markers of inflammation.* For detailed discussions of these types of test and their conceptual background, we refer the reader to the specialized literature, in particular to the reference lists in Chapters B.5, B.6, B.7, C.1, C.2, and C.4 of *Klinische Liquordiagnostik* by Zettl et al. (2003, 2005).

Granulocytes and Activated Forms of the Lymphocytic Series

Granulocytes possess a distinct morphology in May–Grünwald–Giemsa–stained preparations of the CSF, and *neutrophilic* and *eosinophilic* granulocytes are practically always unequivocally identifiable (see Fig. 3.1). Most CSF neutrophils have a *segmented nucleus.* In the acute inflammatory phase, if the cytological preparation is processed immediately after lumbar puncture, most of these cells will actually be seen to have a *hypersegmented nucleus,* with up to six segments and easily discernible bridges between them. Neutrophils with a *band-shaped nucleus* are also readily identifiable but constitute no more than 1 % of the total neutrophil population.

The phagocytosis of pathogens, other noxious influences, and commencement of antibiotic treatment cause the neutrophils with a segmented nucleus ("segmented neutrophils") display progressively more marked features of degeneration as the illness progresses into its next phase (the remission phase). The bridges between the nuclear segments disappear, while the segments themselves become fragmented and fuse together, creating "spherocytes" that contain small nuclear fragments or a single large fragment (see the many illustrations in the following section).

The eosinophilic granulocyte nucleus has essentially the same morphology as the segmented neutrophil nucleus, except that it usually possess no more than three segments, sometimes without any recognizable bridges between them. The cytoplasm of these cells contains characteristic rust-colored granules. Their functional properties (phagocytosis, modulation of cellular and humoral immune processes) come into play predominantly in cases of parasitic infection (particularly with nematodes), in some types of mycosis, and in allergic, hypersensitivity, and foreign-body reactions (certain medications, surgically implanted prostheses). When eosinophilic granulocytes are activated, their nuclear segments become reduced in number and fuse (just as in neutrophil activation), but the cytoplasmic granules remain intact for a longer time and continue to serve as an identifying feature of these cells.

Basophilic granulocytes are rarely found in an inflammatory CSF picture, and are seen almost exclusively in infants and very young children. Their diagnostic significance is unclear. Basophilic (and eosinophilic) granulocytes do, however, become more numerous in the CSF at the beginning of a blast phase of chronic myeloid leukemia. Segmented basophils are roughly the same size as segmented neutrophils, but their segmentation is often less pronounced, perhaps better described as lobulation (sometimes resembling a clover leaf). The characteristic basophilic granules are found in the cytoplasm.

For an adequate understanding of the large subject of *lymphocyte activation* and the *role of lymphocytes in inflammatory reactions* (whether systemic or confined to the nervous system), the CSF cytologist should have the basic knowledge outlined below. Up-to-date information on these topics can be found in Chapters A.7, B.2, and C.1 in Zettl *et al.* (2003, 2005), which we highly recommend. The concepts to be mastered include:

- Basic principles of cellular and humoral immunity.
- Differentiation pathways of the lymphatic stem cell of the bone marrow in the *antigen-independent* phase in the *primary* lymphatic organs, by way of *pre-T and pre-B cells* to mature *T lymphocytes* (in the thymus) and to *multiple determinants* of mature *B lymphocytes* (in the "bursa equivalent," i.e., bone marrow, spleen, and liver), and the migration of these cells to the *secondary* lymphatic organs (spleen, lymph nodes, tonsils, appendix).
- Antigen-induced differentiation processes of *mature B lymphocytes* (*antigen-dependent* phase) to *plasma cells,* which represent the *final* stage of B lymphocyte activation, or to *memory B lymphocytes* (quiescent, mature cells with an immune memory that can be recruited again for another, quicker response at some later time), and the simultaneously active mechanisms for the expression and release of antigen-specific *immunoglobulin antibodies.*
- Special features of the processes of local lymphocytic differentiation and proliferation, and of the immune response, in the central and peripheral *nervous systems,* particularly with respect to the *cerebral barrier systems* (blood–brain, blood–CSF, and blood–nerve barriers) and the *migration of activated lymphocytic populations.*

This basic knowledge will make clear that the *activated forms of lymphocytes* seen in *inflammatory diseases* in CSF cell preparations stained with the May–Grünwald–Giemsa technique (previously known as *lymphoid cells,* a term that is sometimes still used today) actually represent *stages in the differentiation of B lymphocytes,* ranging to the final stage, i.e., the plasma cell. In the classical cell picture, activated lymphocytes with so many types of structure and staining pattern are encountered that the CSF cytologist will certainly be *unable to classify them all specifically* and will, at most, be able to give only a rough *description of their predominant structural and functional type.* This information is usually all that can be obtained from classical CSF cytological examination in inflammatory disease, complementing the findings of the *initial battery of routine CSF testing* which consists of the cell count, routine biochemistry, and culture. The specific classification of activated lymphocytes is necessary only in special cases and requires further, directed immunocytological testing (see Chapter 1, Role of Practical (Classical) CSF Cytological Examination in the Overall Spectrum of CSF Diagnostic Studies).

What specific information about the spectrum of *activated lymphocytes* can be extracted by the CSF cytologist from the May–Grünwald–Giemsa cell preparation, and how can this information be used as an aid to differential diagnosis?

CSF lymphocytes are seen in the cytological preparation mainly as spherical cells varying greatly with respect to size, staining, and nuclear and cytoplasmic features. They are usually less than 25 μm in diameter, although multinucleated forms may be larger. The plasma membrane is smooth and usually sharply demarcated. The nucleus is peripherally located and round or slightly indented. The cytoplasm is lightly or intensely (sometimes very intensely) *basophilic,* and of variable amount. (In an earlier, purely descriptive classification, activated lymphocytes were divided into five categories—small or large lymphoid cells with bright or dark cytoplasm, and lymphoid plasma cells.) A *bright perinuclear area* (archoplasm, Golgi apparatus) may be entirely lacking (in blast forms) or else present to a lesser or greater extent.

These features serve to distinguish activated lymphocytes from nonactivated ones, as already discussed in Chapter 2 (Lymphocytes and Monocytes) and illustrated in Figure 2.**3**, and as shown in Figure 3.**2a, b.** Furthermore, for didactic purposes, we have shown activated monocytes in Figure 3.**2b, c,** and in Figure 3.**3** for comparison with activated lymphocytes; Figure 3.**2c,** also shows a binucleated plasma cell and mitotic divisions of activated lymphocytes. The cytological images in the following section cover a wide range of clinical applications. The activated lymphocytes depicted in these illustrations are recognizable as such and readily distinguishable from activated monocytes. They therefore permit *cytological confirmation* of the suspected diagnosis of an *inflammatory* (*possibly infectious*) *disease of the nervous system.*

A more detailed classification of activated lymphocytes into *subtypes* is much more difficult, because the relation between the cells' visible structure and their functional state cannot always be discerned. One type of cell for which this relation is evident, however, is the *blast progenitor cell,* which exhibits strong basophilia in a relatively narrow area of peripheral cytoplasm, a high ratio of nuclear to cytoplasmic area, and a mostly spherical, usually centrally lying nucleus, *unaccompanied* by any perinuclear structures.

The distinction between *CSF plasma cells* and the other types of activated lymphocytes seen in inflammatory diseases of the nervous system is a difficult matter, as CSF plasma cells differ morphologically in a number of ways from their more readily identifiable counterparts in the bone marrow and peripheral blood. Plasma cells in the bone marrow and peripheral blood are relatively easy to recognize by their large cytoplasm (low nuclear-to-cytoplasmic ratio), an eccentrically placed, oval nucleus with clumped chromatin (suggesting a hub-and-spokes pattern), and a perinuclear area that is only faintly seen, if at all. Plasma cells in the CSF, however, rarely match this description. Their cytoplasmic vesicles are much less numerous and less prominent. They often possess a *large perinuclear area* occupying a *marked indentation of the nucleus,* and they may be *multinucleated.* These features may aid in the cytological identification of CSF plasma cells, but with respect to nuclear structure, nuclear-cytoplasmic ratio, and cytoplasmic basophilia their morphology differs little from that of other cell types in the practically continuous spectrum of activated lymphocytes (and their transitional forms) and thus provides no definitive identifying clues. A just discernible perinuclear area is also a feature of activated lymphocytes, but the accompanying nuclear indentations are less prominent and may be absent. Occasional mitoses and multinuclearity (Fig. 3.**2c** and Fig. 3.**37a, b** later) indicate increased cell proliferation and/or a disturbance of the process of cell division.

Cytoplasmic basophilia is not a reliable criterion for the identification of activated lymphocytes or plasma cells, for two reasons. On the one hand, on immunocytochemical staining some lymphocytes lacking this feature will exhibit marked immunoglobulin synthesis. On the other hand, plasma cells in which antibody production has waned or ceased may display only weak cytoplasmic basophilia and a barely discernible perinuclear area. The morphological differences between CSF plasma cells and their counterparts in the bone marrow and peripheral blood, which were described in the previous paragraph, can only be explained as the result of differences in function (see Zettl *et al.* 2003, 2005).

The wide morphological variation of activated lymphocytes and plasma cells in the classical CSF cytological picture, including many transitional forms, is to be understood as reflecting an underlying diversity of function. We will sum up the present discussion by observing that any attempted subclassification of this heterogeneous group of cells with a common stem cell origin may be a largely arbitrary exercise without any real benefit for differential diagnosis. We therefore recommend grouping all such activated lymphocytic forms in the CSF (when the activation is due to *inflammation,* rather than neoplasia) under the collective term *activated lymphocytes.*

Fig. 3.**1** Left: neutrophilic granulocytes in bacterial meningitis with marked hypersegmentation. Right: eosinophilic granulocytes with varying degrees of segmentation, from ventricular CSF. Center: an activated monocyte and a lymphocyte.

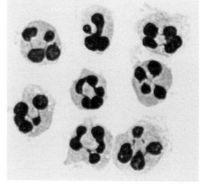 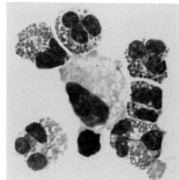

Fig. 3.**2** Lymphocytes in various states of activation (i.e., stages of differentiation).

a Stages of differentiation ranging from nonactivated (first column on the left) to activated lymphocytes and plasma cells of increasing size and with increasing basophilia of the cytoplasm, as well as formation of nuclear indentations with a perinuclear (Golgi) apparatus. The first column on the right has plasma cell progenitors.

b Another array of lymphocytes in progressively more advanced stages of differentiation from the left to the right, ranging to plasma cells, similar to **a**. Two monocytes are shown in the first column on the right to enable comparison of cell size and shape.

c Activated lymphocytic cells (middle column) differentiating into plasma cells. Compare these with the monocytes in the right column. The left column has binucleated plasma cells undergoing mitosis (prophase and anaphase).

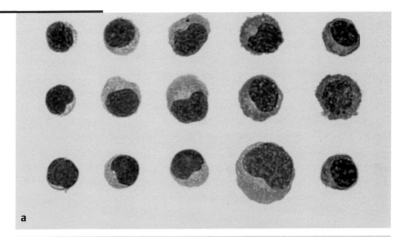

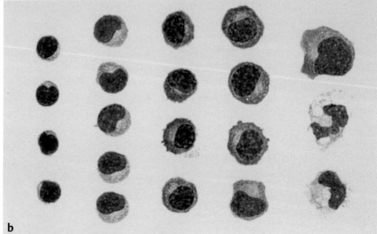

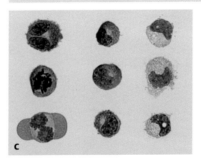

Fig. 3.**3** Juxtaposition of activated lymphocytic cells (upper row) with mildly activated monocytes of varying nuclear and cytoplasmic structure (lower row).

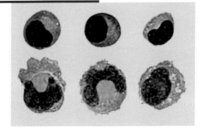

Cytological Findings in Infectious and Inflammatory Diseases

The findings of CSF cytological examination with May–Grünwald–Giemsa staining in infectious and inflammatory disease follow a *typical triphasic course*:

- The initial *polynuclear* (*neutrophilic, granulocytic*) *phase* is characterized by a nonspecific reaction, triggered by chemokines and lymphokines, which manifests itself as granulocytic pleocytosis. It occurs when the blood–brain and blood–CSF barriers are invaded by pathogenic organisms of practically *any* type, but its quantitative and temporal course varies, depending on the organism. In some diseases, e.g., viral meningitis, the polynuclear phase may have ended by the time the initial diagnostic lumbar puncture is performed.

- The ensuing *mononuclear* (*lymphocytic/monocytic*) *phase* is characterized by a marked reduction of both the cell count and the granulocyte fraction. In this *reactive phase*, beginning 3–5 days after the initial polynuclear phase, lymphocytes and their activated forms become prominent, as an expression of an *immune response*, while monocytes and their activated forms play the role of *phagocytes* for the removal of cellular and tissue debris, and the pathogenic organisms themselves (cf. Chapter 4).

- In the final *humoral* or *reparative phase*, the elevated cell count and the mainly mononuclear cellular picture gradually return to normal. Rare activated forms of monocytes and lymphocytes, representing residual cellular activity in the wake of infection, can sometimes be found in this phase for relatively long periods of time.

The length of these phases varies depending on the etiology and pathogenesis of the infectious process, in addition to other factors. The precise temporal course of the cytological abnormalities is usually *typical* of a group of disease processes without being *specific* for any single disease, i.e., it can be used to narrow down, but not to pinpoint, the differential diagnosis. Important factors affecting the cytological picture include the *type of pathogen*, the *site* of the infectious process, its *route of entry*, the *timing of the initial lumbar puncture* from the onset of symptoms, the *age* of the patient, and the *stage of the disease in its course* (complete remission, chronic recurrent process, chronic phase), as well as the nature and timing of the *treatment* provided.

1. The triphasic course of the CSF cytological picture is clearly seen in patients with *purulent bacterial infections* (meningococci, pneumococci, streptococci, *Listeria, Haemophilus influenzae*, etc.). In such patients, CSF obtained by lumbar puncture *within 24 hours of the onset of symptoms* generally has a cell count exceeding 1000 cells/μL. The granulocyte fraction is 85–99 % in the initial polynuclear phase. If antibiotics have already been given before the lumbar puncture, the cell count and granulocyte fraction may both be considerably lower, with a greater percentage of lymphocytes and monocytes (increased mononuclear phase). *Listeriosis* often has an encephalitic component, which creates a mixed polynuclear and mononuclear cytological picture in the CSF. A marked granulocytic picture in the initial phase of listeriosis is illustrated in Figure 3.**10**.

2. In *nonpurulent bacterial infections*, an *exclusively* granulocytic phase is seen rarely, if ever. In the early stage of *neurotuberculosis*, granulocytes may indeed be the predominant cell type in the CSF, but they represent a diminishing percentage of CSF leukocytes as the treatment takes effect. For a long time thereafter, a *mixed picture* prevails, in which lymphocytes are often the main cell type, with more than 5 % activated lymphocytes and plasma cells. (Immunocytochemistry reveals B lymphocytes that synthesize IgA and, less frequently, IgG.) A typical example is shown in Figure 3.**16**.

   In *neuroborreliosis*, the granulocyte fraction in CSF from the initial lumbar puncture is usually very low. The CNS infection manifests as an abnormal, *mononuclear* cytological picture, in which *lymphocytes* predominate and the fraction of activated lymphocytes and plasma cells may be as high as 25 %. (Immunohistochemistry reveals B lymphocytes positive for IgG, IgA, and IgM; IgM is usually the predominant type.) *Neurosyphilis* is associated with a *mixed picture*, mainly mononuclear (lymphocytes, activated lymphocytes, plasma cells), but consisting of rare granulocytes as well.

3. Mixed pictures with lymphocytic predominance are also found in a number of rarer diseases—*neurobrucellosis, leptospirosis, Legionnaires disease*, CNS infection with *Mycoplasma pneumoniae*, and *Whipple disease*.

   In *fungal infections* (candidiasis, cryptococcosis, aspergillosis, etc.), the early CSF picture may be either mainly granulocytic or mixed, with activated lymphocytes and plasma cells. In the chronic stage, lymphocytes predominate.

   The cellular picture in *protozoal infections* is either mainly lymphocytic, with activated lymphocytes and plasma cells (toxoplasmosis, including when it occurs as an opportunistic infection in acquired immune deficiency syndrome [AIDS]; cerebral malaria), or else mainly granulocytic (amoebic meningoencephalitis).

   Parasitic infections of the nervous system produce either a lymphocytic or a mixed picture. *Eosinophilic granulocytes* are a rare finding in neurocysticercosis, but they are commonly seen in toxocariasis and trichinosis.

4. In *viral infections* of the nervous system, the cellular picture of the CSF takes a triphasic course, just as it does in bacterial infections, but the *quantitative* aspects of the three phases are markedly different. The initial cell count is usually well under 1000 cells/μL, and a *purely* granulocytic phase, if it does occur, is of no more than brief duration. Pure granulocytosis is thus an uncommon finding in the CSF obtained in the initial lumbar puncture, which, in most cases of viral infection, is not performed until a few days after the onset of cerebral signs and symptoms. Instead, the initial finding is usually a mainly lymphocytic picture, with a granulocyte fraction well under 20% (see Figs. 3.**25**–3.**31**, 3.**36**, 3.**37a**). As the secondary mononuclear phase proceeds, the granulocyte fraction rapidly declines (except when the infection has an encephalitic component), whereas the fraction of lymphocytes and their activated forms increases until the immune system succeeds in fighting off the infection, whereupon clinical remission begins and the lymphocyte fraction diminishes once again. The fraction of monocytes and their activated forms varies according to the need for these cells to perform their phagocytic function. Because the cellular picture is relatively uniform across a wide variety of viral infections, we will not list the different kinds of viral pathogen here in great detail. We will merely describe the special characteristics of two types of viral infection.

Early summer meningoencephalitis (ESME) can be distinguished from neuroborreliosis by its mainly *granulocytic* cellular picture at the onset of symptoms, which then changes relatively rapidly to a mainly lymphocytic picture.

In *human immunodeficiency virus (HIV) encephalopathy*, the CSF cell count rarely exceeds 30 cells/μL and the cell picture is mainly lymphocytic with activated forms, unless other opportunistic infections of AIDS are simultaneously present (e.g., other viral diseases, toxoplasmosis, neurotuberculosis, mycoses) and produce their own characteristic CSF cell picture. In one case of *combined HIV encephalitis and generalized necrotizing* Toxoplasma *encephalitis,* reported by Tumani (Neurology Department, University of Ulm, Germany), the CSF cytological examination revealed protozoa in the *tachyzoite* stage, which were present not only intracellularly in both granulocytes and monocytes, but also extracellularly (tachyzoites are also called trophozoites or endozoites). With the author's permission, we have reproduced two illustrations from this report (Fig. 3.**39a**, **b**). In AIDS-associated *cryptococcosis*, the pathological CSF abnormalities are less extensive than in cryptococcosis in HIV-nega-

tive individuals. Another noteworthy feature of HIV encephalitis is that the cellular immune response weakens as the chronic disease takes its course (cerebral infection with HIV alone, in the absence of other pathogens, is associated nearly exclusively with activated B lymphocytes of the IgG type; thus, when IgA and IgM types are also found, a concomitant opportunistic infection is almost certainly present.)

5. The cellular picture in inflammatory disorders of the nervous system *in which no pathogenic organisms can be found,* such as *autoimmune diseases* and other conditions, is described in Section C.1 of the text by Zettl *et al.* (2003, 2005).

6. Secondarily triggered *reactive pleocytosis* is caused by a *foreign body* that induces an inflammatory reaction in the CSF. The "foreign body" may consist of extraneous material that has been inserted, for example, into the lumbar theca; on the other hand, it may consist of particulate or soluble matter derived *from the patient's own body,* but of a type or types *not normally found in the CSF.* Reactive pleocytosis can thus be caused by a hemorrhage, traumatic brain injury, or brain tumor impinging on the CSF space—here the "foreign bodies" are erythrocytes, brain parenchymal cells, and tumor cells or their fragments, respectively. Likewise, an irritative cytological picture in *ventricular* CSF may result from a reaction (material intolerance) to a ventricular drainage catheter, manipulative injury to the ventricular wall (during neurosurgical operations, or by vigorous or excessive CSF withdrawal during puncture), or the presence of cell fragments within the ventricles. Finally, reactive pleocytosis can be produced by certain intrathecally administered antibiotics, immunosuppressive medications, and immune modulators (drug-induced meningitis).

7. In chronic inflammatory diseases of the CNS, and in intracranial processes of many types that are accompanied by an inflammatory reaction, certain nonspecific, reactive cell types may be found in the CSF, most commonly multinucleated giant cells, possibly of histiocytic, i.e., of monocytic, origin. These reactive forms are capable of phagocytosis (cf. Chapter 4), but we have chosen to illustrate them in this chapter (cf. Figs. 3.**40**–3.**57**), because they predominantly indicate the presence of an inflammatory process. For diagnostic purposes, it is important to distinguish these multinucleated forms from Langhans giant cells (Fig. 3.**49**), which may signal the presence of tuberculous meningitis (evidence of "caseation" in the cytoplasm).

Inexperienced examiners are liable to *misdiagnose* highly polymorphic, heavily stained reactive giant cells as *neoplastic* giant cells. To facilitate this important distinction for differential diagnosis, we have provided illustrations of singly and multiply nucleated giant cells from malignant brain tumors in Figures 3.**58**–3.**61**. For further illustrations of tumor giant cells in comparison with transitional, premalignant forms, and for their distinction from individual, reactive giant cells, see also Chapter 5.

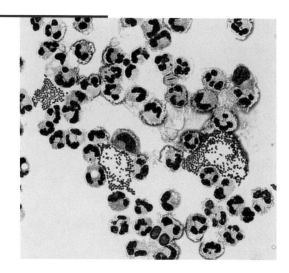

Fig. 3.**4** Acute bacterial meningitis—polynuclear (granulocytic) initial phase. Meningococci, mainly extracellular, are seen. There is incipient phagocytosis in a few granulocytes, mostly in the upper left part of the image.

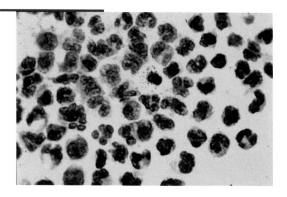

Fig. 3.**5** Bacterial meningitis with markedly altered neutrophilic granulocytes. In the center is a degenerated granulocyte with phagocytosed diplococci. Marked nuclear degeneration is seen, indicating the beginning of remission. Rare monocytes are also seen.

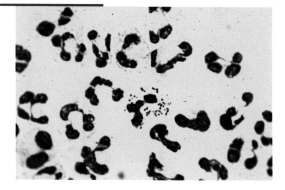

Fig. 3.**6** Polynuclear initial phase of bacterial meningitis. In the center is a granulocyte with phagocytosed diplococci. Granulocyte hypersegmentation indicates toxic cell damage.

Fig. 3.**7** Bacterial meningitis in the early remission phase. The illustration shows granulocytes with phagocytosed meningococci (lower right corner; [arrow]); mononuclear cells in various stages of activation, with partly vesiculated cytoplasm; and occasional erythrocytes and activated lymphocytes.

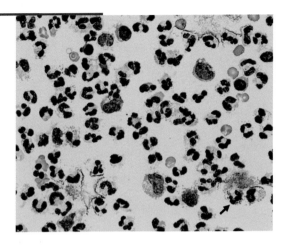

Fig. 3.**8** Bacterial meningitis in the early remission phase. The illustration shows numerous granulocytes, some of which are altered; occasional spherocytes and erythrocytes; rare granulocytes with phagocytosed meningococci; and several activated monocytes.

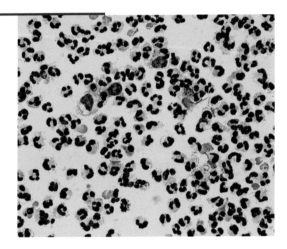

Fig. 3.**9** Remission phase of bacterial meningitis. The illustration shows hypersegmented, altered granulocytes with diplococci. Two monocytes in different states of activation and an eosinophilic granulocyte (arrow) are also seen.

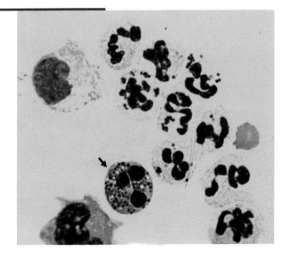

Fig. 3.**10** Acute *Listeria* meningitis (polynuclear initial phase) with rare mononuclear cells and an activated monocyte.

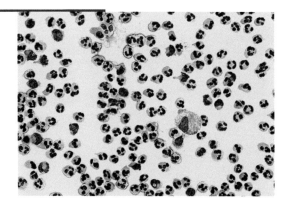

Fig. 3.**11** Bacterial meningitis in the remission phase with predominantly hypersegmented granulocytes, activated monocytes, normal lymphocytes, and one markedly activated lymphocyte.

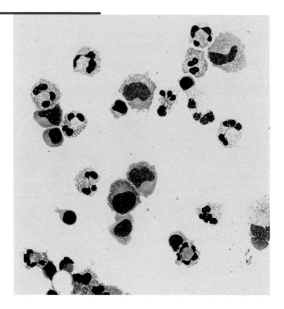

Fig. 3.**12** Late remission phase of bacterial meningitis: hypersegmented granulocytes, some of which still show evidence of cell damage. Endothelium-like cellular aggregates with mononuclear cells separating at the edges are also seen; these mononuclear cells are differentiating into potential phagocytes (see Chapter 4).

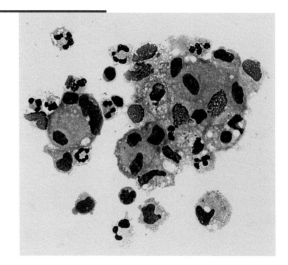

Fig. 3.**13** Late remission phase of bacterial meningitis with predominantly mononuclear cells of diverse sizes and with variously shaped nuclei (activated monocytes, activated lymphocytes). Note: The light cytoplasmic vacuoles in activated monocytes (phagocytosis of lipids?).

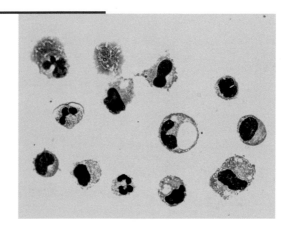

Fig. 3.**14** Eosinophilic meningitis in an allergic reaction. Hypersegmented nuclei in eosinophils and rare monocytes (arrows) are seen.

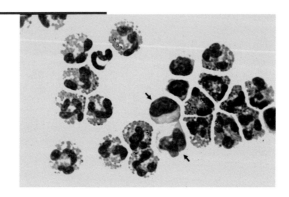

Fig. 3.**15** Remission phase of eosinophilic meningitis with eosinophilic granulocytes and phagocytic cells. There is a leukophage on the left containing phagocytosed eosinophilic granulocytes.

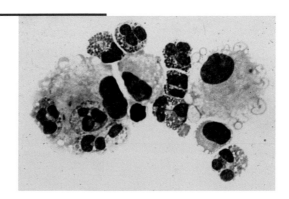

Fig. 3.**16** Acute phase of tuberculous meningitis with hypersegmented granulocytes, activated lymphocytes, and some plasma cell progenitors (arrow); Note the intense basophilia.

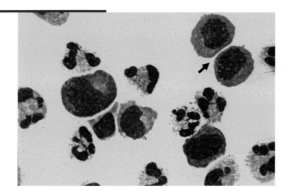

Fig. 3.**17** Mononuclear phase (secondary phase) during remission of *Escherichia coli* meningitis (the polynuclear initial phase had entered remission 6 days after onset).

a Lymphocytic-monocytic cell picture with cells in various stages of differentiation after the end of the initial polynuclear (granulocytic) phase.

b Cell picture 1 week later: monocytes in various states of activation, some in an endotheliumlike arrangement and others separate, with strongly dispersed cytoplasm and an irregularly contoured cell membrane ("signet ring storage form").

c Cell picture 2 weeks after **b**: mononuclear cells of various sizes (activated lymphocytes, activated monocytes) displaying variation in nuclear size and shape and in cytoplasmic components. In comparison with **b**, there is a greater degree of lymphocytic activation.

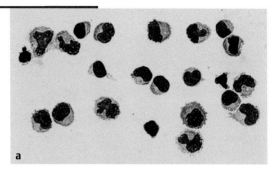

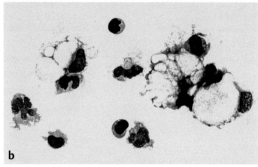

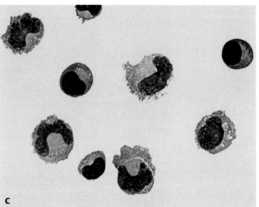

Fig. 3.**18** Mononuclear secondary phase (lymphocytic phase) of cerebral syphilis with predominantly small lymphocytes containing small amounts of lightly stained cytoplasm, as well as two plasma cells.

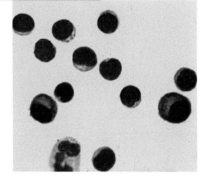

Fig. 3.**19** Cell pictures in neuroborreliosis (Lyme disease).

a Secondary phase of borreliosis with predominantly immune-competent cells in various stages of maturation, ranging to plasma cells; occasional activated monocytes (note the distinction between activated monocytes and activated lymphocytes/plasma cells) are also seen.

b Mainly immune-competent cells of various types and sizes in a case of neuroborreliosis. Note the bipolar mitosis in a plasma cell (arrow).

c Meningoencephalitis in neuroborreliosis with a few activated lymphocytes, a blast cell, a mitosis in prophase, and predominating monocytes in various stages of activation. (Note: this is a relatively atypical cell picture for neuroborreliosis.)

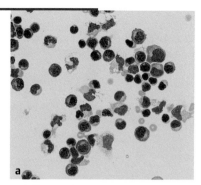
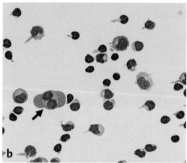
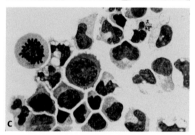

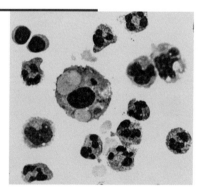

Fig. 3.**20** Granulocytic cell picture in hemorrhagic meningoencephalitis with early monocyte activation, a few lymphocytes, and an erythrophage.

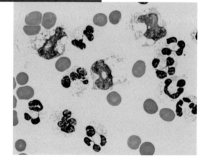

Fig. 3.**21** Granulocytic cell picture indicating reactive pleocytosis after subarachnoid hemorrhage, with activated monocytes, some with apparent lipid storage.

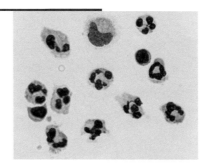

Fig. 3.**22** Granulocytic meningitis as an accompanying manifestation of *brain abscess* (no pathogens could be identified in the CSF). Cell count 30/ μL, 86 % granulocytes, total protein 1425 mg/L.

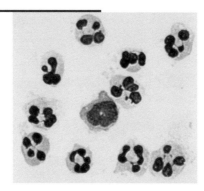

Fig. 3.**23** Reactive pleocytosis in suspected ventriculitis after the resection of a meningioma. Ventricular CSF was obtained postoperatively from an external drainage system. Granulocyte hypersegmentation is seen.

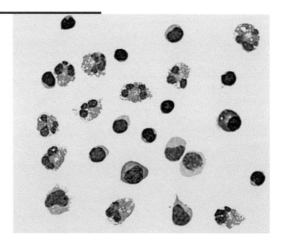

Fig. 3.**24** Eosinophilic reactive pleocytosis in ventricular CSF caused by intolerance to the material of the ventricular drainage catheter that was inserted after brain tumor resection. The cell picture shows eosinophilic granulocytes, lymphocytes, activated monocytes, and a few plasma cells (right). No pathogenic organisms were found.

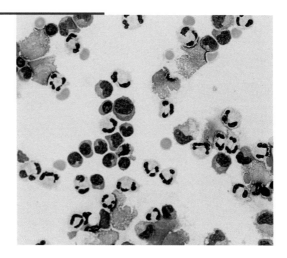

Fig. 3.**25** Relatively acute herpes simplex virus (HSV) meningitis with a still marked polynuclear phase. The cell picture contains activated monocytes and lymphocytes as well as many ghost cells. Artifactual admixture of blood is also seen.

Fig. 3.**26** Relatively acute varicella-zoster virus (VZV) meningitis with granulocytes and, most prominently, activated lymphocytes and plasma cells.

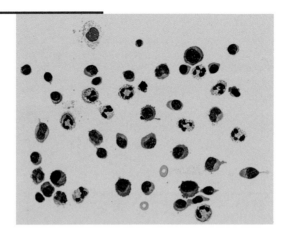

Fig. 3.**27** Subacute viral meningitis (pathogen unknown). The cell picture contains hypersegmented granulocytes, most of which are already altered, as well as two plasma cells and a plasma cell progenitor (arrow) with a hyperchromatic nucleus and marked cytoplasmic basophilia.

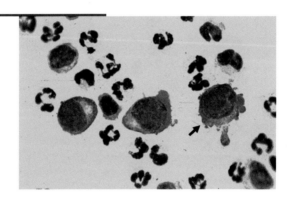

Fig. 3.**28** Viral meningoencephalitis of unknown etiology with large numbers of mononuclear cells, some of which manifest dispersion (breaking up) of their nucleus and cytoplasm. Other findings include hypersegmented granulocytes and lymphocytes in various stages of activation.

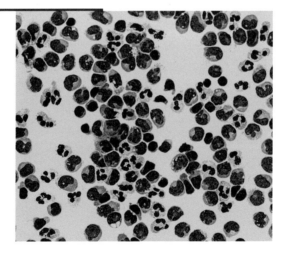

Fig. 3.**29** Relatively acute phase of mumps meningitis with hypersegmented and, in part, altered granulocytes and three hyperchromatic plasma cells, one of which is a polyploid giant cell. At the top are four mononuclear cells in various stages of differentiation (activated lymphocytes).

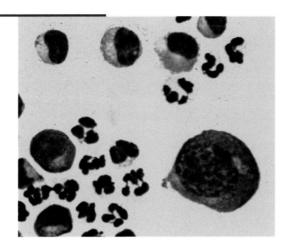

Fig. 3.**30** Relatively acute phase of viral meningitis with degenerated granulocytes, activated lymphocytes, and plasma cells.

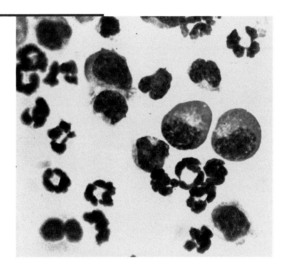

Fig. 3.**31** Relatively acute viral meningitis with granulocytes, two plasma cells, and one plasma cell developing into a "mulberry cell" (arrow).

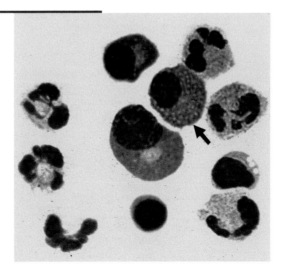

Fig. 3.**32** Mononuclear secondary phase of mumps meningitis. The picture is dominated by immune-competent cells in various stages of activation (mostly mononuclear, with one binucleated cell) undergoing differentiation to plasma cells with a prominently visible perinuclear area (Golgi apparatus). Rare activated monocytes are seen, as well as a single mitosis, the latter indicating an elevated rate of proliferation.

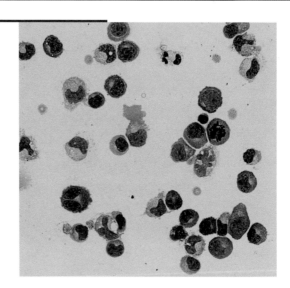

Fig. 3.**33** Enlarged view of CSF cells in mumps meningitis. The picture is dominated by plasma cells with one or two nuclei, in various stages of differentiation and with variable ploidy. Rare lymphocytic degenerated forms are also seen.

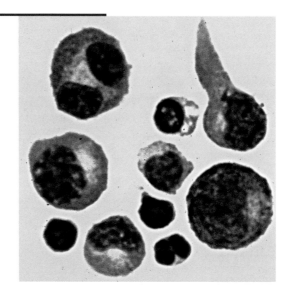

Fig. 3.**34** An illustrative example of VZV meningitis in the mononuclear phase without any activated lymphocytes in the cell picture. The lymphocytes mainly have a clear cytoplasm; some have naked nuclei. There are also rare monocytes and a few erythrocytes (artifactual).

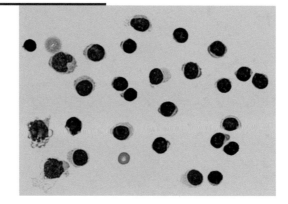

Fig. 3.**35** Mononuclear phase of viral meningitis (caused by rubella virus) with lymphocytic forms in various stages of activation. There are also activated monocytic cells with vesicles. (Note the different appearances of activated monocytic and lymphocytic forms.)

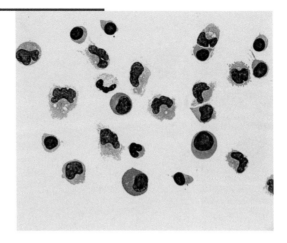

Fig. 3.**36** Enlarged view of CSF cells in viral meningitis in a phase that is still partly granulocytic. Two plasma cells with different nuclear structures and cytoplasmic components are seen; in the older nomenclature, these plasma cells would have been designated as reticular (upper plasma cell, arrow) and lymphoid (lower plasma cell, arrowhead). At the top is a storage cell of the "mulberry" type.

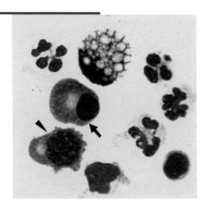

Fig. 3.**37** Two cases with multi-nucleated plasma cells.

a Enlarged view of CSF cells in relatively acute viral meningitis: plasma cell with four nuclei and perinuclear clearing, and two activated monocytes with lobulated nuclei. Artifactual admixture of blood is also present.

b Trinucleated plasma cell with nuclei of different sizes in acute viral meningitis (the erythrocytes are an artifact of lumbar puncture). Note the nearly complete fusion of the cleared perinuclear areas adjacent to the three nuclei.

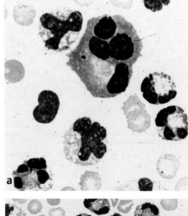

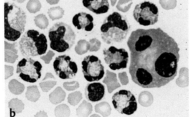

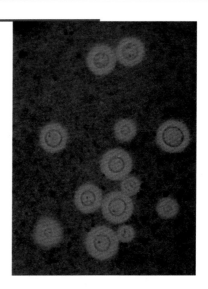

Fig. 3.**38** India ink preparation of CSF from a patient with cryptococcal meningitis (caused by *Cryptococcus neoformans*). There is a mixed cell picture consisting of granulocytes, lymphocytes and their activated forms, and activated monocytes. (Image courtesy of Professor Pfister, Medical Microbiology, Friedrich Schiller University, Jena, Germany.)

Fig. 3.**39** Part of the cell picture in a patient with human immunodeficiency virus (HIV) encephalitis combined with opportunistic *Toxoplasma* encephalitis with intra- and extracellular *tachyzoites* (pictures kindly from Tumany, see text).

a highly enlarged view of a granulocyte with one intact tachyzoite and another in the process of division (arrows). Adjacent to it are a noninfected granulocyte and a few activated lymphocytes.

b Left: a granulocyte containing three tachyzoites (arrows). Adjacent to it is a degenerated activated monocyte and below is a degenerated granulocyte. Right: a monocyte containing tachyzoites in the process of division (broken arrow). An extracellular tachyzoite is clearly seen at the top, whereas the object in the bottom left is probably an extracellular tachyzoite undergoing degeneration (arrowheads).

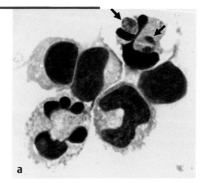

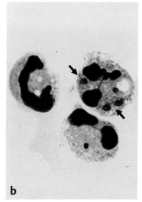
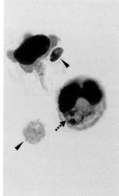

Fig. 3.**40** Cytological images in giant cell meningitis of uncertain etiology. No evidence of malignancy was found at autopsy (Sayk and Wieczorek).

a An undifferentiated giant cell with polyploid, chromatin-rich nucleus containing a large nucleolus. The cytoplasm is basophilic with vacuoles seen at its outer edge. Hypersegmented, somewhat altered neutrophilic granulocytes are also present.

b A multinucleated giant cell with nuclei with an unusually distinct structure and large nucleoli. Note the irregular contours of the plasma membrane. Granulocytes with degenerative changes and one hyperchromatic plasma cell are also seen.

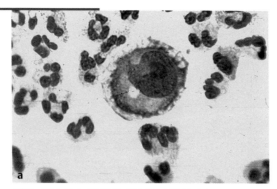

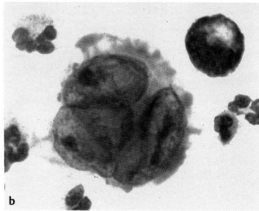

Fig. 3.**41** Cluster of cells with mono- and polynuclear cell forms (probably of histiocytic origin) in different stages of activation. A giant cell is forming; at the periphery cells are separating and beginning transformation to phagocytes. Degenerated granulocytes are visible in the upper right.

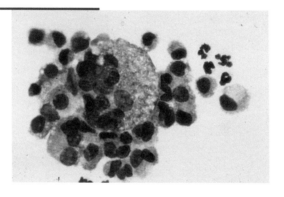

Fig. 3.**42** Further transformation of a polynuclear giant cell which is beginning to separate from a cluster of cells (probably of histiocytic origin). In the two components of the cell cluster directly under this giant cell, other giant cells are in the process of formation.

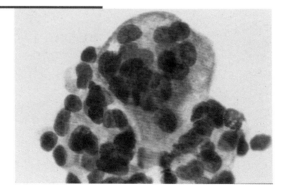

Fig. 3.**43** Terminal differentiation of a foreign body giant cell which is beginning to separate itself from a cluster of cells (probably of histiocytic origin). Vacuoles in the cytoplasm indicate lipophagocytosis.

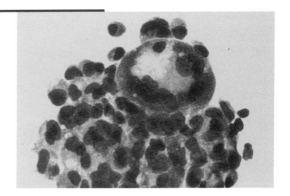

Fig. 3.**44** Ventricular CSF after brain surgery. Center: terminal differentiation of the polynuclear cell to a lipophage. Some of the variably activated mononuclear cell forms surrounding the central cell (probably of histiocytic origin) are also undergoing similar terminal differentiation. A few of these are in the process of separating themselves from the cluster.

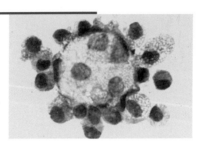

Fig. 3.**45** Polynuclear storage cell with peripherally located nuclei. Adjacent to it there are mononuclear progenitor cells (probably histiocytes) in an early stage of transformation. The erythrocyte (lower right) provides an indication of size.

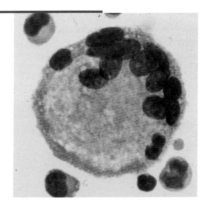

Fig. 3.**46** A phagocytic polynuclear giant cell with a nearly even distribution of the nuclei in the cytoplasm which has a dispersed and finely granular appearance.

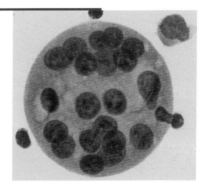

Fig. 3.**47** Polynuclear foreign body giant cell with an entirely peripheral distribution of nuclei. Note the dispersed cytoplasm with areas of increased density, basophilia, and vacuolation, especially in the periphery.

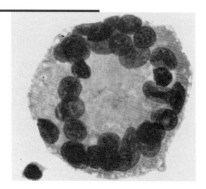

Fig. 3.**48** Multinucleated foreign body giant cell as a special reactive cell type associated with ventricular drainage. The nuclei are diffusely dispersed in the cytoplasm. There is evidence of amitotic division and the cytoplasm is lightly basophilic with many vesicular inclusions (phagocytosis).

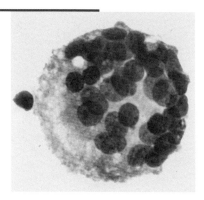

Fig. 3.**49** Multinucleated Langhans giant cell (exclusively occurring) in tuberculous meningitis with accompanying hemorrhage. Some of the nuclei have amitotic extensions; the cytoplasm is homogeneous, acidophilic ,and lightly basophilic at the periphery. Cell fragments are seen next to the giant cell. The erythrocytes provide an indication of size.

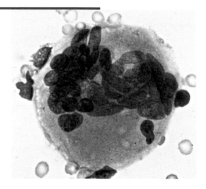

Fig. 3.**50** Loose cluster of degenerated cells with a multinucleated giant cell. The periphery of the giant cell is vacuolated.

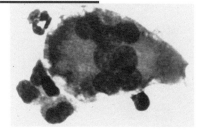

Fig. 3.**51** Deeply stained multi-nucleated giant cell in meningoence-phalitis, with nuclear dissolution and release of nuclear chromatin, as well as cytoplasmic vacuolation typical of a cell in apoptosis.

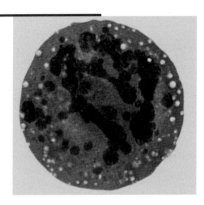

Fig. 3.**52** Multinucleated giant cell with phagocytosis of nuclear chromatin and lipid material (heavily vacuo-lated, lightly basophilic cytoplasm). Note
the large nucleoli. There is evidence of amitotic division of the nuclei (increased number of nuclei).

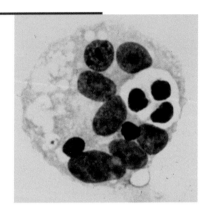

Fig. 3.**53** Multinucleated foreign body giant cell with large vacuoles. The vacuoles are comparable in size to the neighboring mononuclear activated cells and deformed granulocytes.

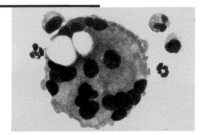

Fig. 3.**54** Giant storage cell in mitosis (prophase); some of the mononuclear cells adjacent to it (probably histio-cytes) are partly degenerated, others are in varying stages of activation.

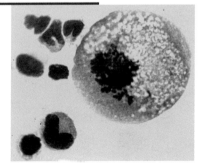

Fig. 3.**55** Multinucleated foreign body giant cell with giant vacuole (lipid phagocytosis?), giving the misleading impression of a signet-ring cell, with adjacent sessile and activated mononuclear cells (probably histiocytes).

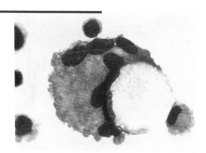

Fig. 3.**56** Multinucleated storage cell containing large amounts of phagocytosed material derived from degenerated cells. The erythrocyte at the left is for scale.

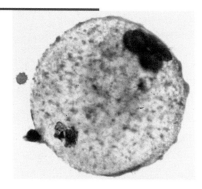

Fig. 3.**57** Macrophage cluster (reactive pleocytosis) with a giant signet-ring cell in the CSF from a patient with a severe brain contusion. Markedly deformed granulocytes are applied to the surface of the signet-ring cell.

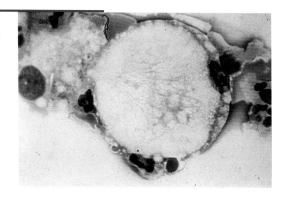

Fig. 3.**58** Acute hemorrhage in metastatic hypernephroma. In the upper part of the picture, there is a still largely undifferentiated cell complex, possibly of endothelial origin, becoming activated to macrophages (arrow). In the epithelial (lower) part of the picture, there are separated, mononuclear, hyperchromatic cells containing vacuoles and brownish-green–tinted cytoplasm (amorphous hemosiderin?). These findings suggest possible malignant degeneration; immunocytochemical marker tests are indicated.

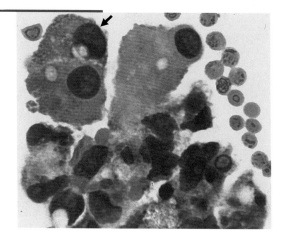

Fig. 3.**59** Multinucleated giant cell with large nuclei and nucleoli, a markedly abnormal nuclear-to-cytoplasmic ratio, and intensely basophilic cytoplasm. Adjacent to it are small, partly degenerated cells (tumor suspect cells). As there is a high degree of suspicion of malignant degeneration, immunocytochemical marker tests are indicated.

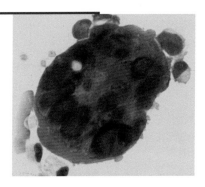

Fig. 3.**60** Highly polyploid mononuclear tumor giant cell in meningeal sarcoma. The erythrocytes provide an indication of the scale.

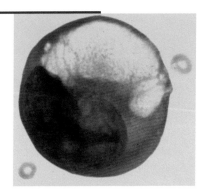

Fig. 3.**61** Highly polyploid mononuclear tumor giant cell with deformation of its chromosomal structure: pathological mitosis in prophase or tumor cell in early apoptosis.

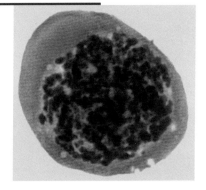

4 Pathological CSF Cell Findings in Intracranial Hemorrhage and Traumatic and Hypoxic-Ischemic Brain Injury

H. Kluge, V. Wieczorek, O. W. Witte, E. Linke, K. Zimmermann, M. M. Kluska, S. Isenmann

Intracranial hemorrhage and traumatic and hypoxic-ischemic brain injury induce a variety of cellular responses. The major question posed to the cerebrospinal fluid (CSF) cytologist generally concerns the *macrophage populations* capable of phagocytosis of blood cells that have entered the subarachnoid space or tissue cell fragments that are anomalously present within it. The information of greatest importance to the clinician is whether the CSF *contains hematomacrophages,* i.e., *erythrophages, hemosiderophages, leukophages,* and mixed forms.

The experienced CSF cytologist will have little difficulty identifying these macrophage populations in the traditional May–Grünwald–Giemsa cytological preparation. These clinically important types of cell are described in this section and illustrated in Figures 4.**1**– 4.**37**.

An understanding of the *cellular origin* of the various types of macrophage is essential background knowledge for the CSF cytologist, even if it is not the primary object of clinical interest. We will therefore briefly summarize current knowledge in this area.

The entry of blood and cellular degeneration products of brain tissue into the CSF spaces as the result of the above-named pathological processes causes, in the *initial phase,* an acute, *nonspecific foreign body reaction.* In this reaction, intense *leptomeningeal irritation* manifests itself as an elevated granulocyte fraction with beginning activation of local monocytes derived from the blood (*reactive pleocytosis*). Its intensity depends on the severity of the precipitating injury.

The *disposal (clearing) phase* first becomes evident in the CSF about 6–10 hours after the primary event. *Activated mononuclear cells* begin to appear at greater frequency, either individually or in loose clusters; these cells are predominantly activated monocytes and histiocytes (monocytic origin) but may be activated forms of ependymal/epithelial, or mesenchymal origin (Figs. 4.**2**–4.**9**). Their nucleus is rounded, sometimes indented, eccentrically placed, and occasionally hyperchromatic. Their cytoplasm is homogeneous or dispersed depending on the degree of activation. It contains fine acidophilic granules, and it usually has an irregular border with protuberances and pseudopodia. The activated monocytes or histiocytes are occasionally already engaged in *erythro- and/or lipophagocytosis* at this early stage (Figs. 4.**4**–4.**9**). This is most commonly seen in children in the early phase of hemorrhage into the CSF space.

Erythrophages are the first type of *hematomacrophage* to develop from the activated cells of monocytic origin (see Figs. 4.**1**, 4.**10**, 4.**11**). They appear in the CSF about 8–12 hours after the precipitating hemorrhage (in the literature times range from 8 to 24 hours), rapidly increase in number in accordance with the extent and severity of the hemorrhage, and begin the task of the enzymatic breakdown of hemoglobin. *Hemosiderin,* a product of hemoglobin degradation, appears in the cytological picture about 3–4 days after hemorrhage (2–5 days in the literature). It is visible as brownish-black granules or clumps inside the hematomacrophages, occupying the spaces in between the more or less thoroughly digested erythrocytes, which are often arranged in a gridlike pattern. The macrophages at this stage consist of mixed forms of *erythro-/hemosiderophages* (see, among others, Figs. 4.**12**–4.**16**, 4.**18**, and 4.**20**). These mixed forms are also seen in all cases of recurrent hemorrhage.

Pure *hemosiderophages* appear 4–5 days after a single or multiple hemorrhage and can still be found in the CSF for weeks or even months thereafter (Fig. 4.**29a–c**). Hemosiderin should not be confused with *melanin,* a pigment associated with melanoma and metastases of melanoma in the CNS, which appears *greenish-black* with the May–Grünwald–Giemsa stain (see Chapter 5, Melanoma). The distinction is of obvious importance in differential diagnosis.

Iron-free *hematoidin* (identical to *bilirubin*) is formed in the final stage of hemoglobin breakdown. It is seen as amorphous, brownish-yellow or yellowish crystalline deposits, which can be either intracellular or extracellular after phage autolysis (Figs. 4.**25**, 4.**30**, 4.**31**).

Macrophages or hematomacrophages that have phagocytosed not only erythrocytes and/or hemosiderin, but also *white blood cells,* are called multipotent macrophages (Figs. 4.**18**, 4.**21**, 4.**22**, 4.**25**, 4.**26**). Granulocytes, for example, can be seen within the macrophages, either intact or in the form of spherocytes. Hematomacrophages can also phagocytose tumor cells in the CSF (Fig. 4.**23**).

A finding of erythrophagocytosis and/or hemosiderin in the CSF is reliable evidence that pathological hemorrhage into the CSF space has taken place, but the diagnosis may be problematic if these cytological criteria are not fulfilled. If the cytological picture shows blood in the CSF, reactive pleocytosis, and a larger number of activated monocytes, but no erythrophagocytosis or hemosiderin, fresh hemorrhage into the CSF space can be suspected, and this should prompt further diagnostic testing by imaging techniques (see below). If the CSF cytology shows suggestive, but not definitive, evidence of a subarachnoid hemorrhage and the brain scan is negative, then the CSF cytologist is faced with the problem of determining whether the hemorrhage is an artifact.

The *artifactual* admixture of blood in the CSF is a common and often unavoidable result of lumbar puncture (see the neurological literature and Chapter 2, Lumbar puncture artifacts). If the lumbar puncture yields bloody CSF despite the *absence of clinical suspicion of subarachnoid hemorrhage,* then the physician performing the lumbar puncture should *inform the cytology laboratory* that this is the case, and perhaps also perform a three-test-tube test to provide further evidence of a "traumatic tap." Communication between the physician and the laboratory is of the essence (and should be part of routine practice anyway). The cytology laboratory may have considerable difficulty processing the specimen if it is not told of the bloody tap and receives only a single test tube for analysis. It will be in a much better position to establish a diagnosis if informed, for example, that the CSF became progressively less bloody in the second and third tubes. As long as the conditions detailed in Chapter 1 (Proper Handling of CSF Specimens Before Cytological Examination) are met, it still should be possible for the cytological preparation to be carried out within 2 hours of the lumbar puncture. If the *ratio of erythrocytes to granulocytes* in the cell picture is more or less the same as that in blood, then the occasional finding of erythrocyte aggregates on monocytes *cannot* be considered proof of hemorrhage (cf. Figs. 4.**7**, 4.**15**, 4.**16**). Various auxiliary CSF tests are often said to be useful for the detection or exclusion of hemorrhage, including measurement of the ferritin level and various spectrophotometric methods based on the different spectral properties of hemoglobin, oxyhemoglobin, methemoglobin, and bilirubin. These tests may provide additional information, but a positive result is not necessarily specific for hemorrhage.

We must digress here to comment briefly on the relative diagnostic value of imaging studies and CSF cytological examination in the detection of bleeding into the CSF spaces. It is certainly true that CSF cytological examination, whenever it provides evidence of subarachnoid hemorrhage, still furnishes no information about the source and location of the bleeding (unlike computed tomography (CT) and magnetic resonance imaging (MRI), which might, for example, reveal a ruptured saccular aneurysm). Yet CT and MRI, despite their ever-improving sensitivity, still cannot reveal small amounts of blood in the CSF so well that CSF cytology can simply be dispensed with after a negative imaging study, when the crucial clinical question is, *"Subarachnoid hemorrhage, yes or no?"* CSF cytological examination is the more sensitive test and should therefore be performed *in all cases of suspected subarachnoid hemorrhage when no blood is detected by CT or MRI* (as long as there is *no contraindication to lumbar puncture,* such as anticoagulation, an intracranial mass, or obstructive hydrocephalus). This is especially true later on in the course of subarachnoid hemorrhage, i.e., in the subacute phase and afterward, when blood will have disappeared from the CT image, but cytological examination will still reveal evidence of hemorrhage.

Hematomacrophages often additionally exhibit *lipophagocytosis,* i.e., phagocytosis of lipids derived from cell fragments. The May–Grünwald–Giemsa cell preparation shows phagocytosed lipids as *empty (i.e., unstained) vacuoles* that are usually considerably *smaller* than the phagocytosed erythrocytes (cf. Figs. 4.**15**, 4.**21**, 4.**22**, 4.**25**–4.**28**, 4.**32a, b**). *Pure lipophages* (also known as gitter cells, scavenger cells, or foam cells) can be found in the CSF in *traumatic brain injury, cerebral atrophy,* and *ischemic brain damage,* regardless of the presence or absence of accompanying hemorrhage. Their frequency depends on the extent of the injury and its proximity to the CSF spaces. They are often found in very large numbers in ventricular CSF obtained postoperatively from external ventricular drains. They may be as large as hematomacrophages, or even larger. Sometimes the borders between their vacuoles dissolve and the vacuoles join; in the extreme case, a *signet-ring form* appears, with a peripherally located cell nucleus. (Caution: confusion of these cells with other types of signet-ring cell, e.g., those seen in adenocarcinoma, may lead to an unfounded suspicion of malignancy.)

Vacuolation revealed by May–Grünwald–Giemsa staining actually provides no more than *initial evidence* of lipophagocytosis. Objective confirmation requires *lipid staining,* as shown, e.g., in Fig. 4.**32b**. In practice, lipid staining is rarely necessary to answer the diagnostic questions posed to the cytologist and need not be done as a routine component of cytological examination of the CSF.

Nonhemorrhagic traumatic brain injury, cerebral atrophy, and ischemic brain damage are not the only diseases than can produce a significant elevation of the CSF cell count with a *mainly granulocytic pleocytosis.* A similar cellular picture can be created by *generalized epileptic seizures* and by *acute metabolic-toxic events.* Acute infectious processes, too, must be considered in the differential diagnosis.

On the Origin of CSF Macrophages

Neutrophilic granulocytes ("*microphages*") take up and destroy *small* particles, particularly bacteria, in a *non-specific* fashion. *Macro*phages, in contrast, take up *specific* kinds of *larger* particles (cell fragments or entire cells, foreign bodies, etc.) and become involved in specific *immune reactions* through the *presentation of antigen*. We will say nothing further about micro-phages in this section, in which we consider the question of the origin of CSF macrophages. (Note: the term "bacteriophage" has been put to other uses in molecular genetics, but is still sometimes used in CSF cytology with its traditional meaning—a cell that takes up and destroys bacteria.)

In the older literature, *all* cell populations capable of phagocytosis (originally, uptake of chemical dye-stuffs), whether located in the bone marrow, in the lymphatic tissues, or in other solid organs, were grouped together under the term "*reticular cells.*" This classification in a single large category was based exclusively on the shared *functional* properties of these cells, which were considered to be the precursor cells of all macrophages, including CSF macrophages. The reticular cells together with the vascular endothelial cells were said to constitute the "*reticulo-endothelial system*" (*RES*), which was later expanded into a "*reticulohistiocytic system*" (*RHS*) that also included histiocytes, plasma cells, tissue mast cells, and osteoclasts.

Over the years, increasingly compelling reasons were found to reject the older hypothesis of macrophage origin as imprecise and inadequately supported (see the relevant literature for further information). A new consensus developed that cell populations distributed over multiple organs should not be grouped together into a "system" merely on the basis of a single common feature, e.g., a common function, as was the case for the RES and RHS. Rather, cells can only be said to form a system if they fulfill the *three* criteria of a *common precursor cell, similar structure*, and *common function*. These criteria are largely met by the so-called *mononuclear phagocytic system* (*MPS*), more precisely designated the *monocyte-macrophage system* (*MMS*). All cells of this system are differentiated forms of monocytic origin that can develop into macrophages. Monocytes migrate out of the bone marrow and travel by way of the bloodstream to many different organs, including the various parts of the central nervous system. After reaching their target organs, and under normal (physiological) conditions, some monocytes remain as immature cells and cell groups ("*quiescent precursor cells*"), whereas others become differentiated, depending on local functional requirements, into *macrophages, histiocytes, or microglial cells* (Hortega cells). The monocytic origin of the latter two cell populations has been conclusively demonstrated.

Histiocytes measure about $40\,\mu m$ in diameter and still resemble monocytes in structure: their nucleus is oval or oblong, sometimes lobulated, and usually eccentrically placed, and their cytoplasm is structured, lightly grayish-blue, with scattered reddish areas, and often contains vacuoles and protuberances of variable size. Their classification as cells of *monocytic* origin thus makes sense for morphological reasons as well (cf. Fig. 4.**9**).

Microglia are found throughout the brain parenchyma. These cells move in ameboid fashion; when stationary, they are thin or even rod-shaped ("microglial rod cells" in the gray matter), with a small nucleus and cytoplasmic processes whose size and number depend on the functional state of the cell. *Pathological changes in the local environment* that stimulate phagocytosis (e.g., encephalitis, infarction, etc.) induce microglia to migrate to the site of injury and differentiate into macrophages (foam cells, lipid granule cells, gitter cells). As the microglia differentiate, their protruding processes are retracted, and they take on a more rounded shape. When they appear in the CSF, these macrophages of microglial-monocytic origin display the typical appearance common to all macrophage types on May–Grün-wald–Giemsa staining.

The multinucleated *giant cells* that appear as a *nonspecific response* to various kinds of stimulus, as discussed in the last chapter in the context of infectious and inflammatory processes in the brain, are a further component of the monocyte-macrophage system. They come into being when the pathological process creates an abundance of poorly digestible large particles. Electron microscopic studies suggest that they are probably formed by the fusion of multiple macrophages or their *monocytic* cells of origin (histiocytes), with dissolution of the individual cell membranes, rather than by a proliferation of cell nuclei through amitotic nuclear division.

The question now arises whether some CSF macrophages might arise from *nonmonocytic precursor cells*, in which case our concept of the monocyte-macrophage system would have to be expanded into a *multiple macrophage system*.

Although the *majority* of CSF macrophages are certainly derived from the *monocyte-macrophage system*, clear evidence for the existence of CSF macrophages of *nonmonocytic origin* has, in fact, been available for some time. In cerebral infarcts, for example, there is a marked increase in the number of subendothelial *pericytes*, which are derived from the *mesenchyme*. These connective tissue cells are already well differentiated to serve a specific function in the normal, physiological state; with the introduction of a pathological change in the environment, they are *unipotent* and phagocytose lipids, i.e., they develop into *lipophages* (Cervos-Navarro and Ferszt 1989). They probably enter the CSF as well.

Similarly, the *epithelial/ependymal* cell populations and the neighboring cells of *mesenchymal* origin that line the walls of the CSF spaces clearly behave in a *unipotent* manner when, under pathological conditions, they enter the CSF as single cells or cell clusters and are exposed to an environment that promotes phagocytosis (cf. Figs. 4.**2**–4.**9**). Further study of the derivation and function of these cells requires going beyond routine May–Grünwald–Giemsa preparations to immunocyto-chemical studies of cell differentiation. The current understanding of the ability of already functionally differentiated, but still unipotent epithelial/ependymal and mesenchymal cells to differentiate into macrophages is still incomplete and contains a number of speculations. Our knowledge in this area may be greatly improved if some of the findings of basic research over the past decade, e.g., with respect to the multipotency of *adult* mesenchymal bone marrow stem cells (Pittenger *et al.* 1999), can be applied with success to the study of pathological processes in the brain.

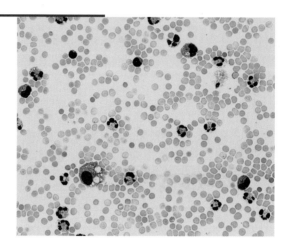

Fig. 4.**1** Acute subarachnoid hemorrhage with early monocyte activation, an erythrophage, and marked reactive pleocytosis.

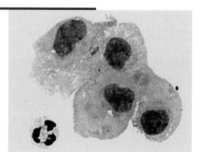

Fig. 4.**2** Cluster of ependymal cells in an early stage of activation and demarcation, transforming into macrophages: the nuclei have clearly recognizable nucleoli and there is evidence of amitotic division. The large, vacuolated cytoplasm, partly acidophilic, partly lightly basophilic, contains granules. Compare the size of these cells with that of the neighboring granulocyte.

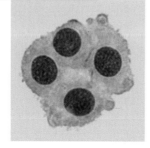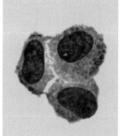

Fig. 4.**3** Cluster of ependymal cells (possibly macrophage progenitor cells). Left: mildly activated cells, still held together in a cluster. Right: early stages of activation and separation from the cluster.

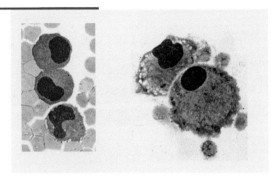

Fig. 4.4 Macrophage progenitor cells of monocytic origin in acute subarachnoid hemorrhage. Left: mildly activated progenitor cells with a hyperchromatic nucleus and finely granulated, acidophilic cytoplasm, beginning to separate themselves from the cluster. Right: strongly activated progenitor cells becoming transformed into macrophages, just about to begin erythrophagocytosis.

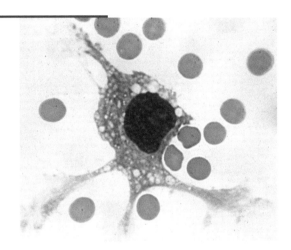

Fig. 4.5 A possibly mesenchymal cell in an early stage of activation to an erythrophage in a patient with acute subarachnoid hemorrhage. The close apposition of the cell to multiple erythrocytes indicates impending erythrophagocytosis. There is marked degeneration of cell processes.

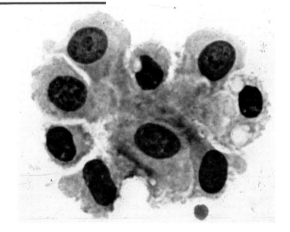

Fig. 4.6 Advanced activation of mononuclear progenitor cells (ependymal cluster) to macrophages in a patient with subarachnoid hemorrhage. The image shows cells in various stages of activation, with a marked tendency to separate from the cluster; erythrophagocytosis is already occurring in the cell on the far right.

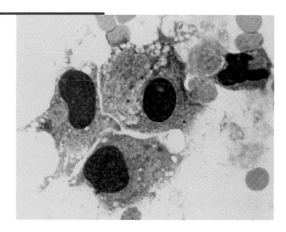

Fig. 4.**7** Progenitor cells (possibly of mesenchymal origin) in various stages of differentiation to erythrophages in a patient with acute subarachnoid hemorrhage.

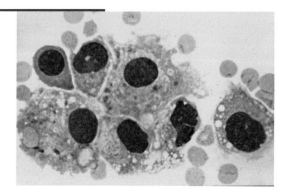

Fig. 4.**8** Cluster of (probably epithelial) cells in various stages of activation and transformation to macrophages in a patient with acute subarachnoid hemorrhage. In the upper left, there is a still undifferentiated precursor cell with markedly basophilic cytoplasm; elsewhere, erythrophages and lipophages can be seen.

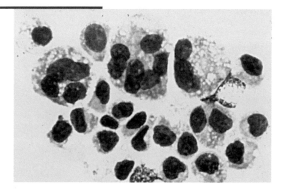

Fig. 4.**9** Macrophage progenitor cells (probably of histiocytic origin) in a loose cluster, some of which are becoming transformed into multinucleated giant cells (top of figure). The cytoplasm of some of these cells is already full of vesicles (lipophagocytosis?).

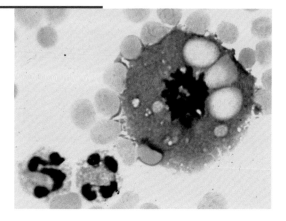

Fig. 4.**10** Erythrophage in mitosis containing erythrocytes in various stages of digestion, in a patient with subarachnoid hemorrhage and reactive pleocytosis.

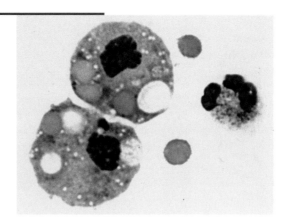

Fig. 4.**11** Erythrophages containing partly digested erythrocytes and vacuolated cytoplasm in a patient with a relatively acute, mild subarachnoid hemorrhage.

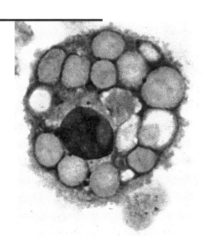

Fig. 4.**12** Erythrophage containing erythrocytes, some still intact, others in various stages of digestion, in a patient with a relatively acute subarachnoid hemorrhage. Hemosiderin granules can be seen in the cytoplasm which has an irregular periphery.

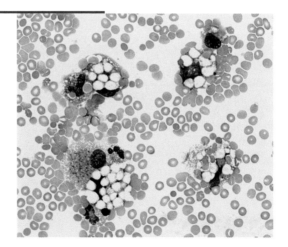

Fig. 4.**13** Erythrophagocytosis in subacute subarachnoid hemorrhage. The phages contain both intact and partially digested erythrocytes (so-called "masked" erythrocytes) as well as hemosiderin granules.

Fig. 4.**14** Erythrophage in ongoing subarachnoid hemorrhage several days after the initial bleeding. with a few intact erythrocytes but mainly digested ones, in a reticulated cytoplasmic grid with hemosiderin granules.

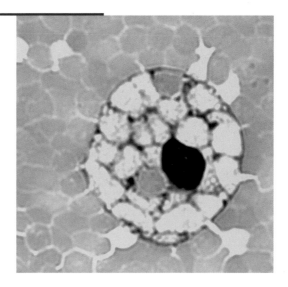

Fig. 4.**15** Various stages in the development of erythrophagocytosis: a small monocyte in an early stage of activation, an erythrophage containing three erythrocytes in different stages of digestion, and a large lipo-hemosiderophage about to phagocytose an erythrocyte (arrow). This cytological exam raises the suspicion of recurrent or older but still ongoing subarachnoid hemorrhage.

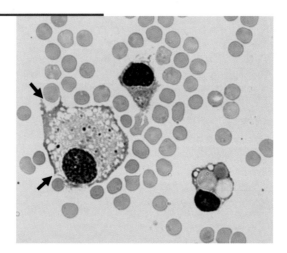

Fig. 4.**16** Macrophage in a patient with a recurrent subarachnoid hemorrhage (i.e., subarachnoid hemorrhage with at least one "re-bleed"). The macrophage contains hemosiderin deposits; it is also about to phagocytose an erythrocyte.

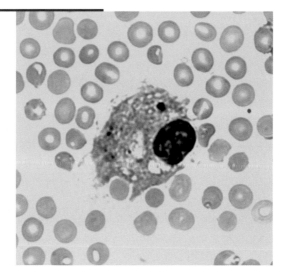

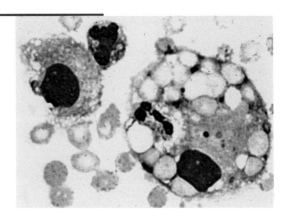

Fig. 4.**17** Remission phase of subarachnoid hemorrhage: a macrophage containing mostly digested erythrocytes, hemosiderin granules, and a granulocyte (erythro-/leukophage), and activated and degenerated mononuclear cells.

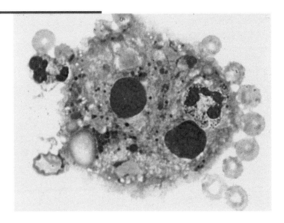

Fig. 4.**18** Binucleated macrophage in a patient with subarachnoid hemorrhage and reactive pleocytosis, containing phagocytosed erythrocytes, a granulocyte, and lipid vesicles ("erythro-/leuko-/lipophage"). Hemosiderin granules can be seen, a product of hemoglobin breakdown (cf. Figs.4.**7**–4.**9**).

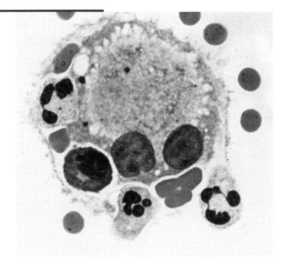

Fig. 4.**19** Binucleated macrophage containing phagocytosed erythrocytes, granulocytes, and a plasma cell in a patient with suspected hemorrhagic meningoencephalitis. Vacuolar storage granules (lipids) and a few hemosiderin granules are also seen in the cytoplasm.

Fig. 4.**20** Binucleated large macrophage (erythro-/hemosiderophage) in a patient with subarachnoid hemorrhage, long after the bleed. This macrophage has a cell membrane and cytoplasm with an interplasmatic, reticulated structure determined by the size of the phagocytosed erythrocytes.

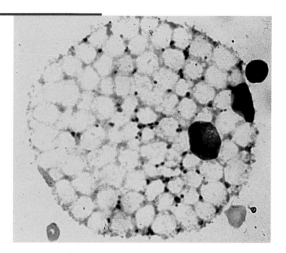

Fig. 4.**21** Two adjacent erythro-/leukophages apparently undergoing separation, with nuclei of different sizes (ploidy and clearly visible nucleoli), in a patient with hemorrhagic meningoencephalitis.

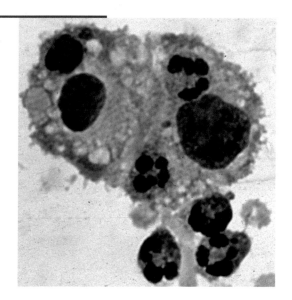

Fig. 4.**22** Macrophage in the late remission phase of meningitis with accompanying hemorrhage, containing phagocytosed spherocytes (easily confused with normoblasts), fragments of leukocytes and erythrocytes, lipids, and hemosiderin granules.

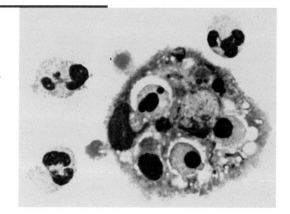

Fig. 4.**23** Erythrophage phagocytosing a tumor cell. The patient had a tumor, tumoral hemorrhage, and eosinophilic reactive pleocytosis after the intrathecal administration of cytostatic agents.

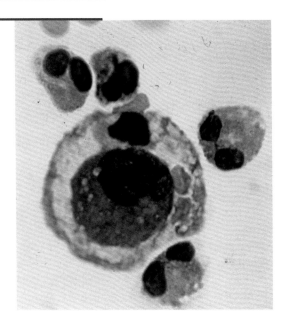

Fig. 4.**24** Late remission phase of subarachnoid hemorrhage with reactive pleocytosis: erythrophage containing digested erythrocytes forming a loose cluster with undifferentiated cells in mitosis that are probably undergoing differentiation to macrophages.

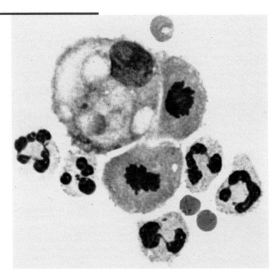

Fig. 4.**25** Complex macrophage cluster with erythro-, sidero-, leuko-, and lipophagocytosis and small hematoidin crystals in a patient with an older, still ongoing subarachnoid hemorrhage.

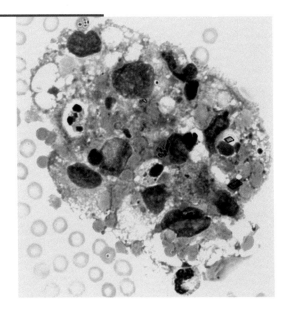

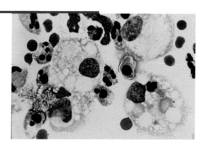

Fig. 4.**26** Cell picture after traumatic brain injury, with erythrocytes, erythro-/lipophages, and granulocytic meningitis. Different stages of spherocyte formation are clearly visible.

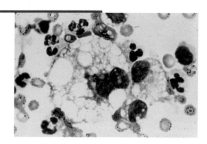

Fig. 4.**27** Subarachnoid hemorrhage and reactive pleocytosis accompanying a brain contusion: binucleated macrophage with inhomogeneous vacuolation, digested erythrocytes, and lipid storage and degradation; adjacent to it is an activated monocyte.

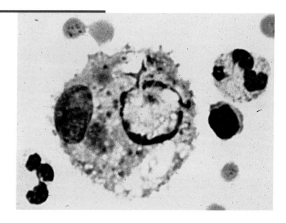

Fig. 4.**28** Macrophage in the late remission phase of *hemorrhagic meningoencephalitis* showing deposition of hemosiderin, lipids, and nuclear chromatin (probably from phagocytosed leukocytes). The neighboring erythrocytes, granulocytes, and lymphocyte provide an indication of size.

Fig. 4.**29** A series of hemosiderophages in the late remission phase of
subarachnoid hemorrhage.

a Hemosiderophages with varying degrees of hemosiderin granulation,
indicating an older hemorrhage.
Compare this cell type with the other cell types present—a lymphocyte,
an eosinophilic granulocyte, and
two activated monocytes.

b An aggregate of hemosiderophages
with varying degrees of granulation
and storage.

c CSF cell picture with mononuclear
and binucleated hemosiderophages
6 months (!) after a traumatic brain
injury. These cells were probably
also engaged in lipophagocytosis.
Compare their size with that of the
nearby erythrocytes (lower left,
upper right).

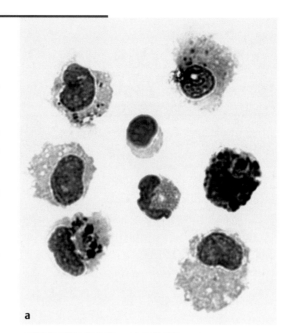

a

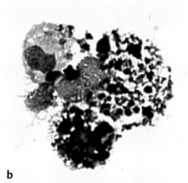

b

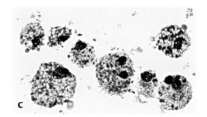

c

Fig. 4.**30** Hemosiderophage containing amorphous and crystalline hematoidin.

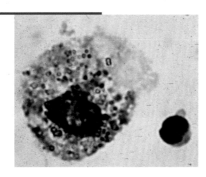

Fig. 4.**31** Hematoidin granules and crystals representing the final stage of hemoglobin degradation after subarachnoid hemorrhage. Left: altered macrophages with amorphous hematoidin granules and small hematoidin crystals. Right: altered macrophage with abundant hemosiderin and two hematoidin crystals, one large, one small.

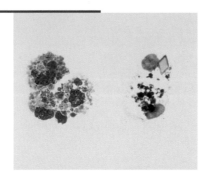

Fig. 4.**32** Lipophages associated with *cerebral infarction*.
a Different developmental stages of monocytes: early activation (lower row) and lipophages (upper row), in a patient with encephalomalacia.
b Left: binucleated lipophage with hemosiderin granules in a May–Grünwald–Giemsa preparation. Right: another binucleated lipophage from the same cell sediment, after Oil Red staining.

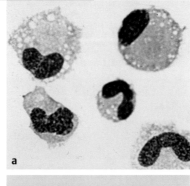

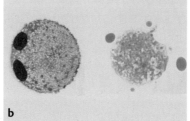

Fig. 4.**33** Multinucleated lipophage with finely and coarsely granulated cytoplasm whose periphery is lightly basophilic and smooth. Note the phagocytosis of erythrocytes by an activated monocyte on the left of the lipophage.

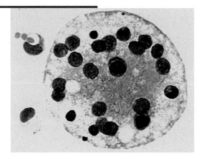

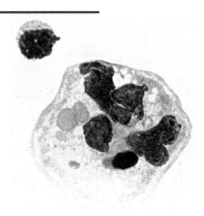

Fig. 4.**34** Multinucleated giant cell, possibly of histiocytic origin, with variably shaped nuclei, after a microhemorrhage. Note the diffuse, lightly basophilic cytoplasm and phagocytosis of erythrocytes and lipids, and storage of nuclear chromatin.

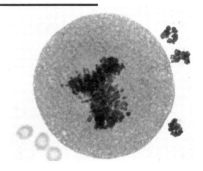

Fig. 4.**35** Giant macrophage in tripolar mitosis in a patient with meningoencephalitis and microhemorrhage. Also seen are erythrocytes and degenerated granulocytes.

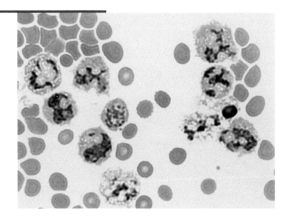

Fig. 4.**36** Bloody ventricular CSF with a suggestion of medication-induced damage to the chromatin within the granulocytes in a patient with ventriculitis. The erythrocytes show hardly any toxic damage.

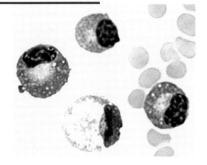

Fig. 4.**37** Plasma cells and a probably lipid-storing signet-ring cell in a patient suspected of having a chronic inflammatory disease of the central nervous system, with accompanying hemorrhage. Note the granulated cytoplasm of the plasma cells, containing small vesicles.

5 Pathological CSF Cell Findings in Primary and Metastatic CNS Tumors, Malignant Lymphoma, and Leukemia

V. Wieczorek, H. Kluge, E. Linke, K. Zimmermann, H.-J. Kuehn, O. W. Witte, S. Isenmann

Fundamentals

Continuous improvement of neuroimaging techniques has made it possible to detect ever smaller tumors of the central nervous system (CNS) and greatly increased the chance of an early diagnosis. Examination of the cerebrospinal fluid (CSF) for tumor cells or tumor-suspect cells is a much less sensitive method of tumor detection, for reasons explained below. Yet, despite the availability of advanced neuroimaging studies, cytological examination of the CSF still retains a useful role in the diagnostic evaluation of brain tumors. Not all types of brain tumor can be detected and reliably assigned to a particular diagnostic category by neuroimaging alone. The evaluation of cellular changes in the CSF in primary and metastatic brain tumors, particularly those that infiltrate the meninges, in the light of our rapidly expanding knowledge in immunocytology and molecular genetics, not only facilitates *diagnosis* but , increasingly often, also provides important information for the choice of an appropriate, specific *treatment strategy*.

Although cytological examination of the CSF is mainly directed toward the detection of tumor cells, or at least of tumor-suspect cells (neoplastic meningitis [or neoplastic meningitis]), it can also provide important additional findings, such as evidence of tumor-related hemorrhage or inflammatory reactions. It is an indispensable method of monitoring the effect of treatment in a number of conditions (leukemia, lymphoma, etc.).

These general remarks will serve as an introduction for the following, more detailed discussion.

The propensity of cells from primary and secondary CNS tumors to *exfoliate* (slough off) and *migrate* in the CSF depends on their *degree of malignancy* (grade), on the *local environmental conditions*, and on *certain limiting factors of the transport pathways*. (Some new information on the mechanisms of these processes and on the target sites for CSF colonization can be found in the current literature in neurology and neuropathology.)

The likelihood of finding tumor cells in the CSF rises if the tumor is *highly malignant* (grade III or higher; rarely, grade II as well), if the *local environment* favors exfoliation and migration into the CSF, and if the *transport* of tumor cells into the CSF is not excessively restricted (e.g., cells derived from metastatic tumor in the brain must be able to traverse capillary systems of those organs that separate them from the CSF). Beside this *triad of important factors*, the *spatial proximity* of an extra- or intracranial tumor to the CSF space is a another, *less important*, determinant of whether tumor cells will appear in the CSF.

It is extremely rare for low-grade tumors near the CSF space to deposit tumor cells in the CSF, although such cells are found somewhat more often after surgical resection of the tumor. Activated forms of non-neoplastic cells can appear as a meningeal reaction to tumors of any degree of malignancy. Thus, the CSF cytologist often faces the task of distinguishing true tumor or tumor-suspect cells from non-neoplastic cells. This problem concerns the diagnosis of low-grade tumors in particular. (This will be discussed further below, as will the relative importance of tumor resection in the context of limiting factors of the transport pathways.)

CSF tumor cells, or at least tumor-suspect cells, are often found accompanying tumors of the following types, if their appearance is favored by the triad of factors mentioned above:

- *Extracranial tumors* can *metastasize* (usually by the hematogenous route, occasionally via the lymphatic vessels) to the leptomeninges, causing *neoplastic (carcinomatous) meningitis*, or to the parenchyma of the brain or spinal cord, leading to the formation of *parenchymal CNS metastases*. On the one hand metastatic disease may be *exclusively leptomeningeal*, i.e., tumor cells may be found in the CSF although no parenchymal metastases are detectable by imaging studies. The vital importance of cytological examination of the CSF in such cases is obvious. On the other hand, tumor cells may also be found in the CSF in *exclusively parenchymal* metastatic disease, unaccompanied by neoplastic meningitis. Cells from a parenchymal tumor can exfoliate and migrate through the choroid plexus and the meningeal vessels into the CSF space, as long as the tumor is highly malignant and the local environmental conditions favor these processes.

■ Exfoliated cells of *primary brain tumors*, as opposed to metastases, are much less commonly found in the CSF. They tend to be seen, if at all, as individual cells or, at most, cell doublets or triplets. Cytological preparations should, therefore, be examined with even more thoroughness than usual when a primary brain tumor is suspected. The experienced CSF cytologist is aware not only of the risk of overlooking evidence of malignancy in such cases, but also of the need to concentrate the CSF cells by sedimentation when the CSF cell count is normal. On the other hand, a large percentage of brain metastases and highly malignant primary brain tumors do ultimately seed the meninges, causing *carcinomatous meningitis*, particularly toward the end of their course. When this occurs, examination of the CSF reveals a marked or severe tumor cell pleocytosis, often accompanied by *reactive pleocytosis* or *hemorrhage*. Sometimes epitheliumlike tumor cell aggregates and tumor giant cells are found as well.

■ Leptomeningeal infiltrates of leukemic cells and malignant lymphoma cells often develop into leukemic or lymphomatous meningitis.

■ Tumors located in the meninges can *metastasize along the CSF pathways*. Exfoliated cells and cell clusters travel through the CSF circulation to distant sites where they grow into new tumors ("drop metastases"). Meningeal tumors are often accompanied by tumor cells in the CSF.

These general principles will be elaborated in further, more concrete detail below in the sections dealing with individual tumor types. The relatively small number of cases studied to date makes it impossible for us to give reliable percentage estimates of the frequency of various CSF findings for each type of tumor. More global estimates, which are not based on classification by tumor type, but rather apply to larger categories of disease, (such as primary versus metastatic, or benign versus malignant brain tumors), can be found in the literature. However, we consider such information to be of limited practical use.

How do the diagnostic capabilities of the CSF cytologist, working with preparations of CSF stained with the May–Grünwald–Giemsa method, compare with those of the neuropathologist, working with specimens of solid tissue?

The *neuropathologist* determines the type of tumor that is present and its degree of malignancy by examining a tissue specimen and carefully taking note of certain distinguishing parameters that, broadly speaking, fall into three classes: *histopathological* (cell density, cellular and nuclear polymorphism, mitotic activity, pathological endothelial proliferation, necrosis of tumor tissue, areas of infiltration), *biological* (molecular genetic, immunocytochemical, and immunohistochem-

ical markers, etc.), and *clinical*. These same parameters also underlie the World Health Organization (WHO) classification of the *degree of malignancy* (*anaplasia*) of CNS tumors into *four grades* (I–IV). Many types of CNS tumor have a clearly definable *histopathological architecture* and are thus easy to diagnose definitively according to such criteria, yet a considerable number of tumor types remain for which this is not possible. The problem is most obvious for tumors in which cells are poorly differentiated to the extent that their distinguishing features are either atypical or else *not specific for any particular tumor type*. In such cases, even if *immunocytochemical markers* (antibodies) are used to detect various tumor cell surface antigens, the neuropathologist will only be able to diagnose an "unclassifiable tumor" or a mixed tumor type.

The CSF cytologist faces much greater difficulties:

■ Tumor cells are found in the CSF as *individual cells* or *very small cell clusters* (only rarely as larger ones). Therefore, the histopathological features of the tumor that are used to define its degree of malignancy and hence its diagnostic classification—that is, the *cell density, pathological endothelial proliferation, necrosis of tumor tissue*, and *areas of infiltration*—are not available for inspection. A tumor cell cluster in the CSF, if present, may be an intact clump of tumor tissue that has separated from a tumor lying near the CSF space; alternatively, it may have been formed by the *secondary aggregation* of tumor cells that were originally present in the CSF as individual cells and then came together under the influence of *local environmental conditions* promoting cell adhesion.

■ Tumor cells in the CSF are also subject to a considerable degree of *secondary change* resulting from the marked *difference between their original surroundings in the tissue and their new, liquid environment*. Although the cells may still be recognizable as tumor or tumor-suspect cells in a May–Grünwald–Giemsa preparation, these changes may render them diagnostically unclassifiable or permit, at most, an assignment to a broad diagnostic category, rather than a specific type of tumor.

■ The distinction between true tumor cells and *nonneoplastic cell types* of similar appearance in May–Grünwald–Giemsa preparations, such as irritative forms of other cell types, incompletely differentiated precursor cells of other cell populations, may also be difficult and necessitate the use of specific marker tests. This problem will be discussed further below.

What combination of criteria can the CSF cytologist still use to diagnose a tumor cell, or at least a tumor-suspect cell, in a May–Grünwald–Giemsa preparation?

■ Unusually or abnormally *large cells*, whose size can vary considerably in a single preparation and among cells of a single type (examples can be found in Figs. 5.**9**, 5.**16**, 5.**17**, 5.**73**, 5.**84**, 5.**96**, and others). Smaller tumor cells may measure 20–25 (μm in diameter, but giant tumor cells of diameter approximately 200(m are not rare, depending on the etiology (see examples in Figs. 5.**19**, 5.**20**, 5.**22**, 5.**23**, 5.**67**, 5.**68**).

- Hyperchromasia, polymorphism, and polyploidy of the *cell nuclei.* The avidity and intensity of nuclear staining is highly variable, depending on the degree of malignancy of the tumor, the vitality of the individual cells, and the extent of degeneration that has already been caused by environmental factors. Tumor cells may have one, a few, or many nuclei, whose *chromatin structure* may be finely or coarsely granulated, clumped, loose, or homogeneous. The cytoplasm often contains ectopic (displaced) pieces of nuclear chromatin, and sometimes also small, round fragments looking like "accessory nuclei" (as seen in Figs. 5.**57**, 5.**72**, 5.**74**). There is often an elevated number of *nucleoli*; these are of variable, and often atypical, size (as seen in Figs. 5.**71**, 5.**72**, 5.**117**).
- An increased number of *pathological mitoses/amitoses* at various stages of division, a few of which are multipolar owing to the polyploid chromosome sets of many neoplastic cells (for illustrations of multipolar mitoses see Figs. 5.**39**, 5.**67**, 5.**87**). Pathological mitoses account for the accompanying findings of nuclear polymorphism and giant tumor cells (Figs. 5.**15**, 5.**23**–5.**25**, 5.**105**, 5.**106**). Giant tumor cells sometimes appear in a form suggesting tumor cell cannibalism or endocytogenesis. In particular, cells of this type are likely to be found after systemic and intrathecal chemotherapy (see Figs. 5.**14**, 5.**101**, 5.**110**).
- The *cytoplasm* of neoplastic cells is markedly or intensely basophilic because it is rich in the RNA components needed for increased protein synthesis. Areas of particularly strong basophilia tend to be found near the cell membrane; in the interior of the cytoplasm, basophilia is often mixed in with, or overshadowed by, cloudlike areas of acidophilia. (See, for example, the gradations of staining in the tumor cell clusters of Figs. 5.**13**, 5.**28**, 5.**38**, 5.**39**, and in the individual cells of Figs. 5.**9**–5.**11**, 5.**15**, 5.**20**, 5.**36**, 5.**37**.) The *cell membrane* or the edge of the cytoplasm can likewise take on many forms: smooth, round, vacuolated with cytoplasmic protrusions, irregular, or punched-out (examples in Figs. 5.**3**, 5.**7**, 5.**18**, 5.**33**, 5.**61**, and elsewhere). In tumor cell clusters, there may be cytoplasmic bridges between cells, and cells at the edge of the cluster are sometimes seen in the process of separating themselves from it (as in Figs. 5.**8**, 5.**13**, 5.**24**, 5.**28**, and elsewhere). *Cytoplasmic inclusions* and *tumor signet-ring cells*, which indicate secretory function,

are often seen in metastases of adenocarcinoma to the brain, yielding a clue to the histogenesis of the primary tumor. The organ and cell type of origin of the primary tumor, cannot, however, be determined with complete precision by cytological examination of the CSF alone (see Figs. 5.**93**–5.**101**, 5.**113**, 5.**114**). Cytoplasmic pigments enclosed in melanin granules are a characteristic feature of melanoblastoma. (For details, see the discussion of this type of tumor, below.)

- Most, but *not all*, tumor cells are characterized by an *elevated nuclear-to-cytoplasmic ratio* (many examples of this can be seen in the illustrations below in the sections on specific types of tumor and are commented on in the accompanying legends).

The classic morphological criteria for tumor cells listed here suffice to enable a "*tumor-cell–typical*" but *not* a "*tumor-cell–specific*" diagnosis. This means that the CSF cytologist will be able to give a *yes* or *no* answer to the basic question *whether tumor or tumor-suspect cells are present*, but they will not be able to reach a more refined diagnosis beyond the broad category of tumor that is present (metastatic adenocarcinoma, melanoma, grade IV astrocytic tumor, malignant lymphoma, medulloblastoma, and leukemia can be diagnosed by experienced CSF cytologists with a high degree of probability, ependymoma less so).

The tumor-cell preparations that are illustrated in the following sections were all examined according the criteria listed above and classified by the neuropathologist's diagnosis of the tumor tissue. Cells that did not satisfy enough of the listed criteria to be unambiguously identified as tumor cells are shown in this atlas with the designation *tumor-suspect cells.* In cases where such cells were found, the figure legend states that immunocytochemical tumor marker tests should be used to confirm the suspicion of neoplasia and establish a precise diagnosis of the type of tumor present.

We have classified the tumor cells shown in the following illustrations in accordance with the *neuropathological classification* and *grading scheme of the WHO, as updated in 2000* in light of new findings in *immunocytochemistry* and *molecular genetics* (Kleihues and Cavenee 2000; Radner *et al.* 2002). Some of the older names of various types of tumor, and earlier classifications, are also used at various places in the text and in the figure legends. For some of the earlier cases in our series, the diagnosis originally reached by the neuropathologist by the then current morphological and histochemical methods may have to be revised if the same tumor was examined with the immunocytochemical and molecular genetic techniques available today. This might well be true of some cases that we have already had to reclassify in accordance with changes in the WHO scheme (as mentioned in the individual relevant sections below). Our basic knowledge in neuropathology and neurooncology is expanding so rapidly that future revisions of the present chapter on CNS tumors will undoubtedly also contain newly updated and more precise diagnoses. Another current source of imprecision is the fact that tumor nomenclature in the neurological and neuropathological literature is not uniform, nor is it completely standardized within either of the two fields. Some redundancies remain to be eliminated, and some gaps remain to be filled (e.g., with regard to spongioblastoma, variants of glioblastoma, and types of sarcoma). Yet, despite these limitations, the May–Grünwald–Giemsa staining method, combined with the criteria described above, still provides a *universally applicable and reliable method* of determining whether tumor or tumor-suspect cells are present—the most important question that the CSF cytologist is required to answer.

An important feature of the current WHO classification, as well as of its predecessor (1993), is that they both dispense with the terms "*primary brain tumor*" and "*secondary brain tumor,*" even though these terms were in use for many years and are still familiar to CSF cytologists from textbooks of neurology.

For the sake of completeness, it should be mentioned that the literature contains reports of tumor cells in the CSF in certain kinds of tumor for which we have, to date, found *no tumor cells at all* or else, in very rare cases, *cells with only a remote suspicion of neo- plasia* in the CSF. In our experience, further study has usually revealed cells of the latter type to be atypical and unclassifiable, rather than neoplastic. We refer the reader to the relevant literature for each of the tumor types for which this is true. *Tumor-suspect cells* have been reported in a few cases of *meningioma* (Dufresne 1972), *anaplastic oligodendroglioma* (Watson and Hajdu 1977), and *neuroblastoma* (Gandolfi 1980). *No* CSF cells with malignant features, but, at most, atypical forms have been reported in *craniopharyngioma* and *neurinoma*.

In view of the limited diagnostic potential of the May–Grünwald–Giemsa method, it is appropriate to ask under what circumstances *immunocytochemical tumor marker tests* are to be considered *necessary, advisable,* or *superfluous* for the purposes of clinical diagnosis and treatment.

- Such tests are *necessary* when a routine May–Grünwald–Giemsa preparation reveals tumor cells or tumor-suspect cells, but the clinical examination, radiological studies, and standard laboratory tests provide *no other evidence* of a primary brain tumor or cerebral metastasis, i. e., in cases of pure meningeal carcinosis. If *definite tumor cells* are present according to the criteria described above, then a full complement of tumor marker studies should be undertaken to determine the tumor type and cell of origin (including a repeated lumbar puncture and testing of the newly obtained CSF for tumor markers), and an interdisciplinary tumor search is also indicated. When *only tumor-suspect cells* are found, tumor marker studies should begin with a *limited search* for the *particular cell populations* that are liable to be *misdiagnosed* as tumor cells (poorly differentiated, *non-neoplastic* precursor cells of meningeal origin, bone marrow cells, irritative forms of the lymphocytic and monocytic series, phagocytes, and *non-neoplastic* giant cell forms).
- Immunocytochemical tumor marker studies are *advisable* when a *primary* CNS tumor is *strongly suspected* but not definitively diagnosed on clinical and radiological grounds, and tumor cells or tumor-suspect cells are found in the CSF sediment. A precise classification of these CSF cells is useful above all in determining the further *treatment*.
- Immunocytochemical tumor marker studies of CSF cells are *superfluous*, in cases of *biopsy-proven primary CNS tumors* and *brain metastases of known source* (including generalized malignant lymphoma with CNS infiltrates), as well as in *leukemia*, which can generally be diagnosed and precisely classified with diagnostic testing of the blood, bone marrow, or both.

We conclude this general introductory section with an important remark: tumor cells or tumor-suspect cells may be present in the CSF in very small numbers, as only a few individual cells or small aggregates. The CSF cytologist will be able to diagnose a tumor (or at least a suspected tumor) from the CSF sediment even though the CSF cell count is *not* elevated above normal. Thus, whenever there is a question of a possible CNS tumor, a CSF sediment should always be prepared and meticulously examined, regardless of the cell count.

Astrocytic Tumors

Astrocytic tumors (gliomas) are epithelial tumors whose most important defining characteristic is the immunocytochemical demonstration of the expression of the *astrocytic intermediate filament GFAP* (glial fibrillary acidic protein) in *tissue specimens*. GFAP expression is used as an *immunocytochemical criterion for tumor classification* (Kleihues and Cavenee 2000; Radner *et al.* 2002; Zettl et al. 2003, 2005) and also provides the basis for the latest WHO classification (2000), in which the astrocytic tumors are subdivided into *pilocytic astrocytoma, diffuse astrocytoma, anaplastic astrocytoma, glioblastoma, subependymal giant-cell astrocytoma* (in tuberous sclerosis), and *pleomorphic xanthoastrocytoma.* These different types of tumor are also assigned a *grade of I–IV,* indicating their degree of malignancy. Pilocytic astrocytoma is a grade I tumor; diffuse astrocytoma, grade II; anaplastic astrocytoma, grade III; and glioblastoma, grade IV, including its variants, giant-cell glioblastoma and gliosarcoma (Kleihues and Cavenee 2000; Radner *et al.* 2002). Classification problems arise because of the existence of numerous mixed types (e.g., oligoastrocytoma with oligodendroglial and astrocytic components, glioneural tumors with astroglial and neuronal components). In such cases, the neuropathologist can reach a reliable diagnosis only with the use of appropriate immunocytochemical marker studies for tumor phenotyping, as described by Wick (in Zettl et al. 2003, 2005), among others. The CSF cytologist must have recourse to the same method, as the differential diagnosis of mixed tumor types is not possible from a classical cytological preparation alone.

In *low-grade* astrocytomas (grades I and II tumors, i. e., pilocytic and diffuse astrocytomas) exfoliation of tumor cells into the CSF is *rare.* Any cells that are found in the CSF can usually be initially characterized only as *atypical* or, at most, *tumor-suspect cells.* Thus, the CSF cytologist can usually do no more, at first, than express suspicion of a tumor. If a precise diagnosis of the CSF cells is required (differentiation from similar-appearing cells of non-neoplastic origin, absence of other evidence of CNS tumor), then the cytologist will need to proceed to an adequate battery of immunocytochemical marker tests for tumor-cell phenotyping. Cytological preparations of the CSF in WHO grade I and II astrocytoma can be seen in Figures 5.**1**–5.**5**.

With regard to pilocytic astrocytoma, a few special points of importance to the CSF cytologist need to be explained here. In the neuropathological literature, one finds statements to the effect that the type of tumor once known as polar spongioblastoma corresponds to what we now call pilocytic astrocytoma. Yet, in the earlier WHO classification of 1993, polar spongioblastoma was assigned to the class of "neuroepithelial tumors of unclear histogenetic origin." The current WHO classification (2000), which we have used as the basis for this chapter, reflects the view that polar spongioblastoma is *not* an independent tumor entity at all, but rather a type of tumor architecture that can be encountered in different kinds of tumor, including gliomas (astrocytoma and others), and even in focal areas of primitive neuroectodermal tumors. The *term* "polar spongioblastoma" was, therefore, eliminated from the WHO's current catalog of tumors in neuropathology. It is still important, however, to distinguish *primitive polar spongioblastoma* as a special entity within the heterogeneous group that used to be called polar spongioblastoma. This very rare, rapidly growing, and *highly*

malignant tumor of childhood is said to be a particular type of tumor on its own. We have seen a case in which the neuropathologist made a probable diagnosis of primitive polar spongioblastoma and we, in turn, found definite tumor cells in the CSF. More precise diagnostic studies were not available at that time, so we could only state that the cells were from a type of astrocytic tumor (see Figs. 5.**28**, 5.**29**). We suspect that the cytological preparations shown in Schmidt's atlas under the heading "spongioblastoma" were, in fact, derived from cases of primitive polar spongioblastoma. Our suspicion is strengthened by the report that one of the patients was a 2-year-old boy (Schmidt 1978, 1987).

In *high-grade* astrocytomas (i. e., grades III and IV), the frequency of exfoliation of cells into the CSF space is much higher, about 10–15 %. The distinction between a grade III and a grade IV astrocytoma cannot always be made definitively even from a combination of histopathologic examination and radiological images, nor can CSF cytology confirm the diagnosis in every case. Thus, in English-speaking countries, the term "malignant glioma" is often used collectively to cover tumors of either grade.

Exfoliated cells from anaplastic astrocytomas (WHO grade III) have markedly malignant features and display tumor-cell morphology. They are characterized by marked cellular and/or nuclear polymorphism and polychromasia, an increase in the size of the nucleus relative to the cytoplasm (elevated nuclear-to-cytoplasmic ratio), and mitoses(Figs. 5.**6**–5.**12**). They can be classified as tumor cells when seen in a May–Grünwald–Giemsa preparation, without the need for any further immunocytochemical testing.

The same is true in almost all cases of *glioblastoma* (also called glioblastoma multiforme), the most common type of *WHO grade IV astrocytoma* (Figs. 5.**13**–5.**18**). These tumors were, at one time, held to be embryonal tumors because of their extremely poorly differentiated appearance. Exfoliated glioblastoma cells in the CSF meet *all tumor cell criteria,* as do cells from the glioblastoma variants *giant cell glioblastoma* and *gliosarcoma* and from *subependymal giant cell astrocytoma* (a separately listed type of tumor). The giant tumor cells shown in Figures 5.**19**–5.**27** were assigned to the correct type of tumor on the basis of their appearance in a classic May–Grünwald–Giemsa preparation alone.

Cytoplasmic polychromasia is seen in CSF tumor cells derived from malignant astrocytomas of WHO grade III, and especially grade IV, and is characterized by usually well-demarcated acidophilic and basophilic areas, of which the former tend to be nearer the cell nucleus and the latter more toward the periphery. The intensity of acidophilia and basophilia varies widely from cell to cell and from tumor to tumor, though, as a rule, heavier intensities are more commonly seen in grade IV tumors. High-grade astrocytomas are often accompanied by inflammatory reactions and hemorrhage.

As the above remarks imply, the unequivocal identification of giant cell glioblastoma and gliosarcoma as types of astrocytic tumor is possible only with the aid of histological and immunocytochemical phenotyping. The classic May–Grünwald–Giemsa cytological preparation is not only insufficient for this purpose, but it also fails to distinguish these tumor types from giant cell sarcoma (Cervos-Navarro and Ferszt 1989). Immunocytochemical differentiation with astroglial and mesenchymal tumor markers has revealed that some giant cell sarcomas are GFAP-positive and thus of astrocytic origin, whereas others are vimentin-positive and thus of mesenchymal origin. It should be noted that we examined the specimens illustrated in Figures 5.**19**– 5.**25** before such methods were available either to us or to the neuropathologists with whom we collaborated. Thus, our final diagnosis of a giant cell glioblastoma was somewhat arbitrary by current standards. Some of these images might perhaps have appeared more appropriately in the section on mesenchymal, non-meningothelial tumors later in the chapter.

The *neoplastic* giant cell types described above can be unambiguously classified as tumor cells, but there are also other, *non-neoplastic* types of giant cell that are *liable to be misdiagnosed* as tumor cells, particularly phagocytic giant cells representing an advanced state of leukocyte activation (differentiation). Tumor marker studies should be done when indicated to reduce the likelihood of this diagnostic error. Examples of nonneoplastic giant cells can be found in Chapter 3 (Figs. 3.**55**–3.**58**).

Pleomorphic xanthoastrocytoma was, until recently, classified as "anaplastic pleomorphic xanthoastrocytoma, WHO grade III." This type of tumor, however, has a more favorable prognosis after resection than grade III anaplastic astrocytoma, and the current WHO classification therefore calls it "*pleomorphic xanthoastrocytoma with signs of anaplasia*," without any numerical WHO grade being assigned. We are not aware of any description in the literature of CSF tumor cells derived from this type of tumor.

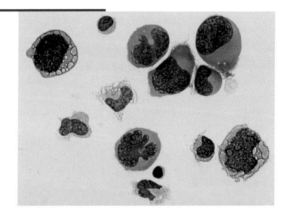

Fig. 5.1 Suspected tumor cells in a patient with grade I pilocytic astrocytoma, characterized by a round or lobulated nucleus with multiple nucleoli; a variable nuclear-to-cytoplasmic ratio; and a partially vacuolated, mostly acidophilic cytoplasm with basophilic areas. Compare the size of these cells with that of the two monocytes (left of center) and the lymphocyte (top). Immunocytochemical studies for tumor markers are indicated.

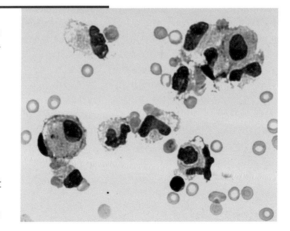

Fig. 5.2 Histologically confirmed grade II astrocytoma. The CSF cytological picture alone arouses *no more than a remote suspicion* of neoplasia. It is dominated by mononuclear reactive forms, probably originating from monocytes and/or ependymal structures. The nuclei are of variable shape with a single nucleolus; the cytoplasm is relatively large with some poorly demarcated areas, which are mostly acidophilic, but sometimes mildly basophilic at the periphery. For comparison, the figure also shows activated monocytes and a lymphocyte. A signet-ring cell is seen in the lower left of the figure. Follow-up examination of the CSF is indicated.

Fig. 5.**3** Uniform cellular reaction in ventricular CSF obtained from an Ommaya reservoir, arousing the remote suspicion of astrocytoma in a 44-year-old man who had a histologically confirmed astrocytoma as a child. The figure shows mononuclear cells with relatively large nuclei, single nucleoli, and a strongly basophilic cytoplasm; these may represent cell types undergoing ependymal or endothelial transformation. Immunocytochemical tumor marker studies are indicated.

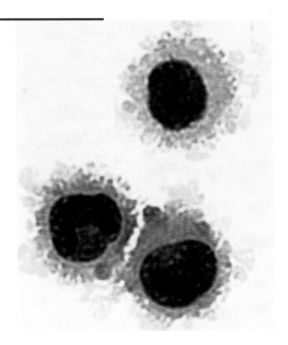

Fig. 5.**4** A cluster of atypical cells in a patient with a histologically confirmed grade II astrocytoma. The nuclei and nucleoli are of variable size, and the basophilic cytoplasm has marked vesiculation. Immunocytochemical tumor marker studies are indicated.

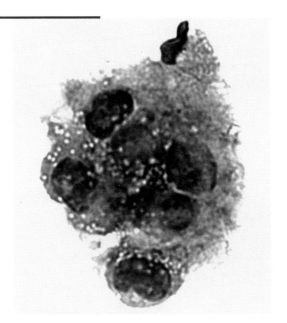

Fig. 5.**5** Markedly basophilic cell (tumor-suspect cell) with a large nucleus, multiple nucleoli, and vacuolated cytoplasm in a patient with grade II astrocytoma. Eosinophilic reactive pleocytosis with activated monocytes is seen. Immunocytochemical tumor marker studies are indicated.

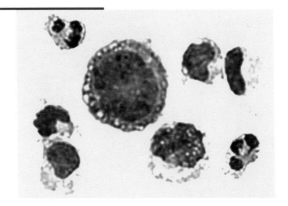

Fig. 5.**6** Cluster of tumor cells in grade III anaplastic astrocytoma, with variable configurations of cell nuclei, nucleoli, and cytoplasmic components. The predominantly basophilic but partly acidophilic cytoplasm has perinuclear vacuolation. There are accompanying pleocytosis and hemorrhage.

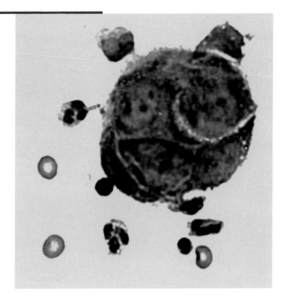

Fig. 5.**7** Mononuclear, polyploid tumor cell in a patient with grade III astrocytoma. The nucleus has multiple nucleoli of variable size; the ring-shaped, strongly basophilic cytoplasm has numerous protuberances. Compare with the surrounding mononuclear cells, some of which are activated, and one of which is apparently beginning to phagocytose an erythrocyte. Accompanying hemorrhage and reactive pleocytosis with eosinophilic granulocytes are seen.

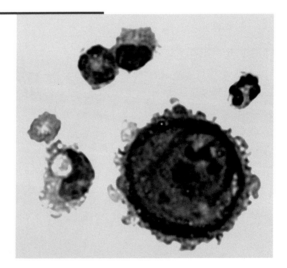

Fig. 5.**8** Cluster of relatively uniformly shaped tumor cells in a patient with grade III astrocytoma. Some of the nuclei are polyploid; many nucleoli are seen, and the cytoplasmic component of the cells is markedly basophilic, although to a variable extent. A mitosis in anaphase/telophase is seen in the bottom right of the figure.

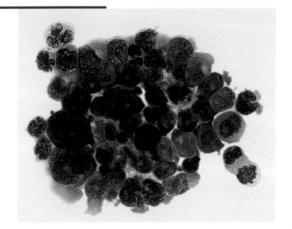

Fig. 5.**9** Tumor cells in a patient with grade III astrocytoma, with conspicuously lobulated, sometimes coarsely structured nucleus. There is marked nuclear polychromasia. The cytoplasm is basophilic with perinuclear clearing. Adjacent to the tumor cells are possible "mini-tumor cells" or small cellular fragments (apoptotic nuclear fragments), some of which are ringed by cytoplasm.

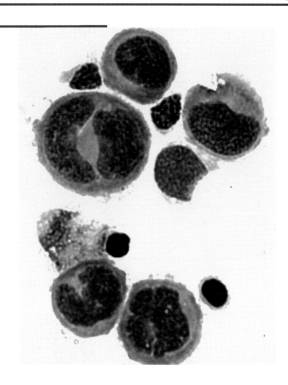

Fig. 5.**10** Tumor cells in a patient with grade III astrocytoma, displaying marked polychromasia and, in particular, basophilia of the cytoplasm. Possible apoptotic nuclear fragments or miniature tumor cells are seen (compare with Fig. 5.**9**). A degenerating signet-ring cell is seen in the top right corner.

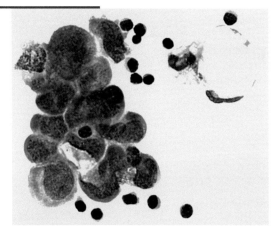

Fig. 5.**11** Cluster of tumor cells of varying size and marked uptake of stain in a patient with grade III astrocytoma. The arrow indicates a degenerating tumor cell of signet-ring type with vacuolated cytoplasm and intracytoplasmic nuclear fragments.

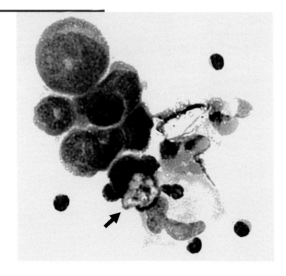

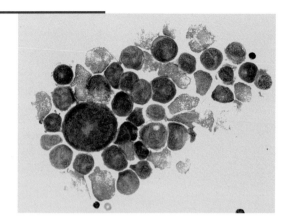

Fig. 5.**12** Loose cluster of tumor cells in a patient with grade III astrocytoma, with a number of small cells and one highly polyploid giant tumor cell with a thin rim of markedly basophilic cytoplasm. Also present are degenerating cells and ghosts.

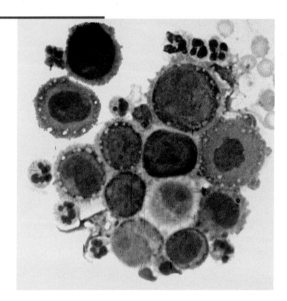

Fig. 5.**13** Neoplastic meningitis in a patient with glioblastoma multiforme, with accompanying hemorrhage and relatively acute reactive pleocytosis. There are numerous polymorphic tumor cells with typical malignant features and variable affinity for stain, predominantly mononuclear; the nucleus has many nucleoli of variable size, and the cytoplasm of some of the cells displays peripheral vacuolation. Pathological mitosis is seen on the right. The granulocytes and erythrocytes provide an indication of the scale.

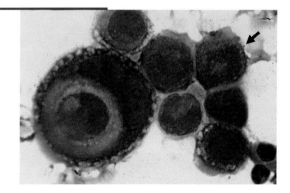

Fig. 5.**14** A cluster of predominantly mononuclear tumor cells, some of which have a poorly defined border between the nucleus and the cytoplasm, in a patient with glioblastoma multiforme. Binucleated giant tumor cell with endocytogenesis, multiple nucleoli, and a vacuolated rim of cytoplasm. There is marked uptake of stain in the nucleus and cytoplasm. Pathological mitosis in prophase is seen (arrow).

Fig. 5.**15** Mononuclear, relatively uniform tumor cells with variable affinity for stain and large nucleoli, in a patient with glioblastoma multiforme. Pathological mitosis in pro-/metaphase in a large tumor cell: chromosome deformation and reticulated cytoplasmic structures are easily seen. The granulocyte provides an indication of the scale. There is evidence of accompanying hemorrhage (degenerating erythrocytes).

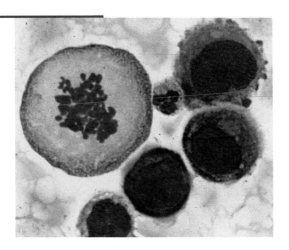

Fig. 5.**16** Relatively uniform, predominantly mononuclear tumor cells in a patient with glioblastoma multiforme. The nucleus is relatively well demarcated from the surrounding cytoplasm. In the center is a multinucleated, polyploid giant tumor cell that contains various structures, some of which are poorly defined. It has a thin rim of basophilic cytoplasm. A pathological mitosis is seen at the bottom right, with abnormal chromosomal division (early anaphase?). The erythrocyte provides an indication of the scale.

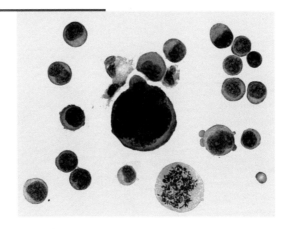

Fig. 5.**17** Overview of relatively uniform, mononuclear tumor cells, some of which are in clusters, in a patient with glioblastoma multiforme. The nuclei are of varying size and shape, and the cytoplasm of variable extent and staining characteristics. Two mitoses in early metaphase are seen (arrowheads), as well as one mitosis in anaphase (arrow).

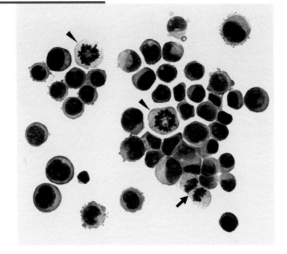

Fig. 5.**18** Tumor cells of variable size and variable nuclear and cytoplasmic structure, some of which are in a small cluster, in a patient with glioblastoma multiforme. The cytoplasmic border is sharp in some cells, and irregular in others, with protuberances. The nuclei are round or oval, there are a few nucleoli, and intracytoplasmic chromatin fragments are seen (arrows). At the bottom is a polyploid giant cell with an irregular nucleus, cytoplasmic protuberances, and broken-off fragments of cytoplasm. A typical signet-ring cell is seen in the cluster (dotted arrow), as is a mitosis in anaphase (arrowhead). The single erythrocyte provides an indication of the scale.

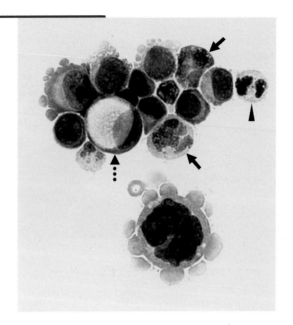

Fig. 5.**19** Tumor cells with three and four nuclei in a patient with a giant cell glioblastoma. The tumor cells have nuclei of variable size and nucleoli, and display evidence of amitoses (arrows). In some places, intracytoplasmic fragments of nuclear chromatin are seen. The cytoplasm has an irregular or smooth border, and is partly acidophilic and partly basophilic. The artifactual admixture of erythrocytes provides an indication of the scale.

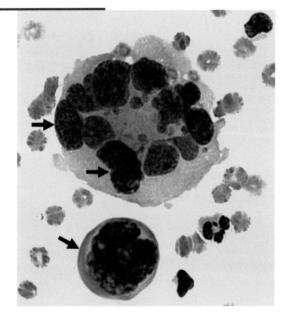

Fig. 5.**20** Highly polyploid tumor cell in a patient with a giant cell glioblastoma. The nucleus is in amitosis (constriction). The tumor cell below it is probably undergoing apoptosis. Artifactual admixture of blood and activated lymphocytes (arrows) is present.

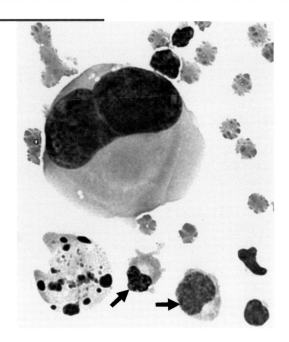

Fig. 5.**21** CSF cytological preparation in a patient with a giant cell glioblastoma showing a cluster of tumor cells of variable size, with a highly polymorphic nucleus and a narrow, strongly basophilic rim of cytoplasm. There are multinucleated giant tumor cells within and adjacent to the cluster (arrows). At the bottom, two signet-ring type cells with large vacuoles show degenerative changes in their nuclei and cytoplasm. The erythrocytes provide an indication of the scale.

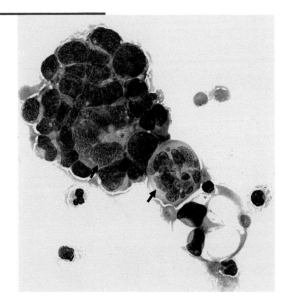

Fig. 5.**22** Mononuclear, highly polyploid giant tumor cell in a patient with a giant cell glioblastoma. The otherwise smooth nuclear membrane is notched at one point (early amitotic division?). The thin rim of cytoplasm is heavily stained and bears fringelike protuberances. A few erythrocytes are also seen.

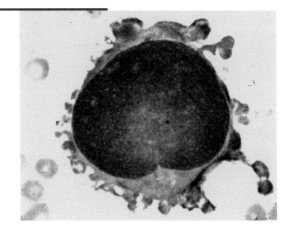

Fig. 5.**23** Highly polyploid giant tumor cell in tripolar amitosis, with nuclei of different sizes (partial separation from cell cluster), in a patient with a giant cell glioblastoma. The narrow rim of polychromatic cytoplasm is of variable depth, and its border is irregular in some areas. Adjacent to the giant tumor cell are other mononuclear and multinucleated tumor cells and a few erythrocytes.

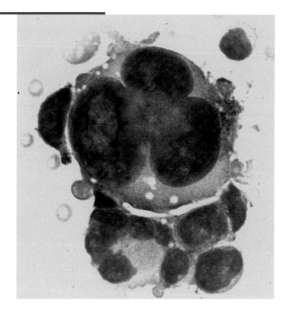

Fig. 5.**24** Loose cluster of tumor cells in a patient with a giant cell glioblastoma. Cells of variable size, some of which are separating from the cluster. Two mitoses in prophase are seen as well as a highly polyploid giant tumor cell in amitotic division (arrow) with thin, deeply stained, irregularly bordered cytoplasmic rim. The erythrocytes are shown for scale.

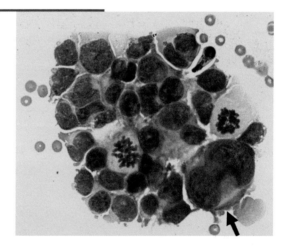

Fig. 5.**25** Giant cell glioblastoma with polymorphic cells. The lumbar puncture was done while the patient was undergoing chemotherapy. A giant tumor cell is undergoing double amitosis. It has a large, partially fragmented cytoplasmic area with markedly basophilic periphery. Apoptotic cells are seen nearby (phagocytosis of nuclear fragments?).

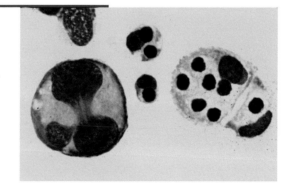

Fig. 5.**26** Giant tumor cell in apoptosis in a patient with giant cell glioblastoma. The erythrocyte provides an indication of the scale.

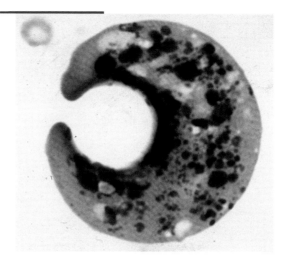

Fig. 5.**27** Apoptosis of a giant tumor cell, and adjacent multinucleated giant cell, in a patient with glioblastoma. The erythrocyte and the monocyte indicate the scale.

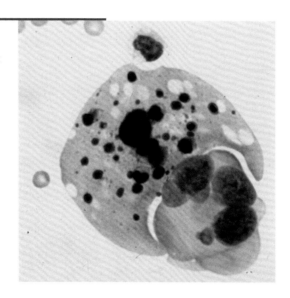

Fig. 5.**28** Probable *primitive polar spongioblastoma* of the cerebellum in a child. This is an independent, highly malignant disease entity (not to be confused with pilocytic astrocytoma). The illustration shows a loose isomorphic cluster of tumor cells, some of which are breaking away from the cluster. The nucleus is variably lobulated with many nucleoli and there is variable expression of malignant features. Some cells exhibit vesiculation of the cytoplasm. Note the nuclear fragmentation and apoptotic generation of extracellular nuclear fragments (arrow).

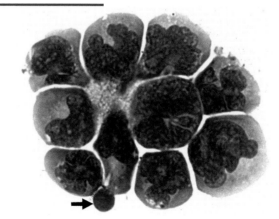

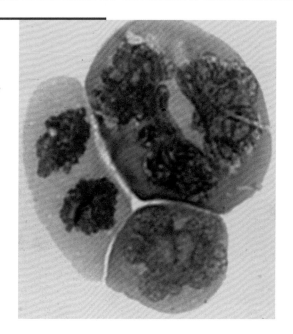

Fig. 5.**29** Tumor cells of variable size breaking away from a tumor cell cluster from the same patient as in Fig. 5.**28**. Note the mitosis in anaphase and possible amitotic division of the highly polyploid giant tumor cell.

Ependymal Tumors

The current WHO classification includes the following types of ependymal tumor: *myxopapillary ependymoma* and *subependymoma* (grade I), *ependymoma* (grade II), and *anaplastic ependymoma* (grade III). Grade II ependymoma has four histopathological variants: cellular, papillary, clear cell, and tanycytic. Grade II ependymoma is distinguished from grade III anaplastic ependymoma by the absence of significant mitotic activity and other anaplastic features.

The cytoplasm of ependymoma cells occasionally contains *glial filaments* that can be revealed by a marker test for GFAP (which is not present in normal ependymal cells). This intermediate type between ependymoma and astrocytoma, called subependymoma, shows a low level of anaplasia. In general, the variants of grade II ependymoma are sometimes difficult to distinguish from low-grade astrocytic tumors, oligodendroglial tumors, and plexus papillomas, forcing the neuropathologist to resort to immunohistochemical marker profiles.

The neuropathological literature describes *ependymoblastoma* as another type of tumor that must be distinguished from anaplastic ependymoma. This type of tumor has a stem-cell character, is assigned WHO grade IV, and is considered to belong to the class of embryonal tumors.

A relatively high percentage of ependymomas is associated with exfoliation of tumor cells in the CSF space. The more anaplastic the tumor, the more likely it is that tumor cells will be seen in the CSF. With lower-grade tumors, isomorphic tumor cell aggregates and loose tumor cell clusters of an epithelial character may be found (Figs. 5.**34**, 5.**35**). The cells in these aggregates and clusters have a small, relatively compact, and eccentrically placed nucleus that contain a single nucleolus and are surrounded by a large, very loose, finely granulated, gray- or light-blue colored cytoplasm. Note that these cells do not possess the elevated nuclear-to-cytoplasmic ratio that often typifies tumor cells. Although readily identifiable, they may display a certain resemblance to lipophages (compare Fig. 5.**35** with Fig. 4.**32a, b**).

Even more conspicuous in CSF cytological preparations, and even more important for diagnostic purposes, are the CSF cells derived from *anaplastic* grade III ependymomas, which have significantly larger, relatively round, and hyperchromatic nuclei, single nucleoli, and a smaller, polymorphic, polychromatic, and vacuolated cytoplasm. The nuclear-to-cytoplasmic ratio is usually shifted toward the nucleus (i. e., elevated), as seen in Figures 5.**31**–5.**33**. There is often evidence of accompanying hemorrhage and reactive pleocytosis.

Fig. 5.**30** Abnormal cellular aggregate in a patient with histologically confirmed ependymoma; large nuclei, nucleoli, and basophilic cytoplasmic protuberances. Compare these cells with the activated monocytes and the two erythrocytes just above them. Immunocytochemical tumor marker tests are indicated.

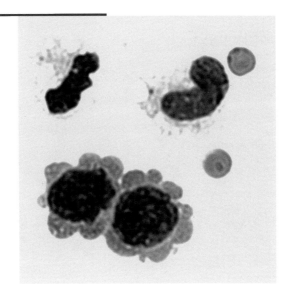

Fig. 5.**31** Tumor cell cluster with polymorphic nuclei and honeycombed, deeply stained cytoplasm (partly acidophilic, partly basophilic), in a patient with an anaplastic ependymoma. The nuclei and cytoplasm exhibit marked degenerative features.

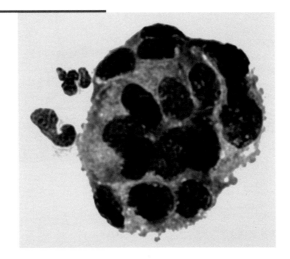

Fig. 5.**32** Mononuclear tumor cell cluster with large, round nuclei and nucleoli of variable size in a patient with histologically confirmed anaplastic ependymoma. The cytoplasm is strongly basophilic; it is a thin rim in some cells, vesiculated in others, with protuberances. Accompanying granulocytic meningitis.

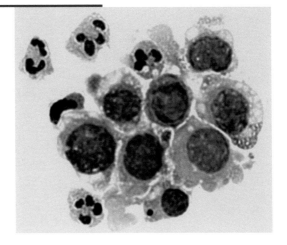

Fig. 5.**33** Polyploid mononuclear tumor cell with markedly loosened, vesiculated, and partly frayed-off basophilic cytoplasm in a patient with an anaplastic ependymoma. There is evidence of accompanying granulocytic meningitis with lack of segmentation of the nuclear chromatin in some cells (arrows) and hemorrhage.

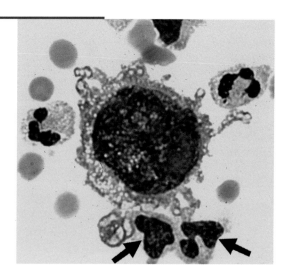

Fig. 5.**34** Cell cluster containing mainly mononuclear tumor cells in a patient with an isomorphic ependymoma. The relatively small, irregularly shaped, compact nucleus has a single nucleolus; the large cytoplasm is markedly loosened and only mildly basophilic. A few smaller tumor cells show increased affinity for stain, indicating a lesser degree of differentiation.

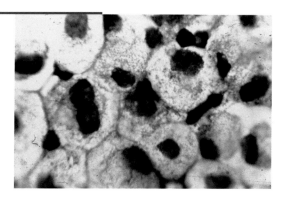

Fig. 5.**35** Tumor cells in a cluster, with a small, coarsely structured, eccentric nucleus and nucleoli, in a patient with an isomorphic ependymoma. The copious, markedly loosened, finely granulated, and lightly basophilic cytoplasm is deeper staining at the periphery.

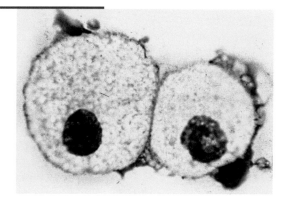

Tumors of the Choroid Plexus

Choroid plexus papilloma and *carcinoma* have a papillary or finely granular surface and float freely in the CSF space except for their attachment to the choroid plexus, which can be either broad based or pedunculated. Occasionally they can also infiltrate the neighboring brain parenchyma or even the dura mater and skull bone. Choroid plexus papilloma, which grows slowly, is classified as a WHO grade I tumor. Choroid plexus carcinoma is classified as WHO grade III.

Plexus tumors tend to produce much more CSF than the normal choroid plexus, sometimes more than can be resorbed by the normal mechanisms. The result of this disturbance in CSF homeostasis is hypersecretory hydrocephalus. The fragile, papillary nature of the tumoral tissue can cause pieces of the tumor to break off; these then travel through the CSF spaces and can give rise to so-called *drop metastases*, which are typically seen in the lumbar theca between the nerve roots of the cauda equina. Accordingly, plexus tumors are relatively frequently associated with a positive finding of cells during cytological examination of the CSF. The iso-

morphic cells and cell clusters of the benign variant of plexus tumor (choroid plexus papilloma) may be difficult to distinguish from the normal cells of the plexus epithelium that can get dislodged into the CSF during lumbar puncture or by other kinds of trauma. Due caution should therefore be used in interpreting findings of this type.

Tumor cells derived from choroid plexus carcinoma tend to appear in smaller or larger clusters in which the peripherally lying cells can often be seen to be separating themselves from the cluster. The cells in these clusters have an epithelium-like arrangement, are mostly isomorphic, and display abnormalities of nuclear and cytoplasmic structure that are typical of tumor cells (hyperchromasia, sometimes polychromasia). A few mitoses can be seen (Fig. 5.**39**). Reactive cells possessing single or multiple nuclei can also appear as an accompanying response to the tumor, complicating the differential diagnosis (Figs. 5.**36**, 5.**37**). The relevant immunocytochemical marker tests will need to be applied in some cases.

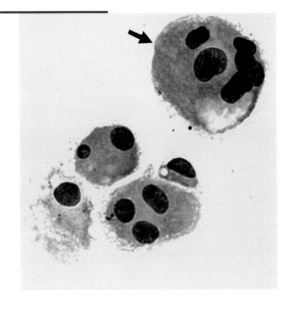

Fig. 5.**36** Atypical cells arousing the remote suspicion of a tumor in a patient with a choroid plexus papilloma: a giant cell (arrow) and mono-, bi-, and trinucleated cells with nuclei of variable size, sharply demarcated from the surrounding cytoplasm, containing nucleoli. Large, finely structured, and lightly basophilic cytoplasm, with vesicular loosening visible in some peripheral areas. Immunocytochemical tumor marker tests are indicated.

Fig. 5.**37** Multinucleated giant cell in a patient with a choroid plexus carcinoma. The cytoplasm is finely structured, irregularly lined, and markedly basophilic with several large acidophilic areas. The cell border is smooth in some places and irregular in others. The nuclei have a single nucleolus. Compare the size of the giant cell with that of the erythrocyte on its left. A foreign-body giant cell is remotely possible and might be considered in the differential diagnosis.

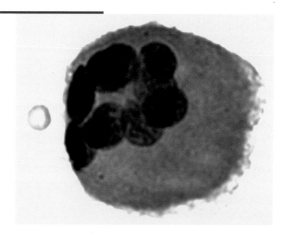

Fig. 5.**38** Cell cluster (broken-off fragment of tumor that has metastasized through the CSF pathways) in a patient with a choroid plexus carcinoma. The relatively uniform tumor cells are arranged in an epitheliumlike pattern. Nucleoli are seen, and the nuclear-to-cytoplasmic ratio is elevated.

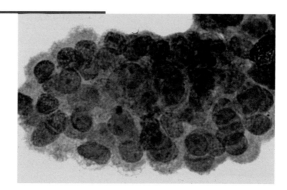

Fig. 5.**39** Tumor cell cluster in a patient with a choroid plexus carcinoma. A multipolar mitosis is seen (arrow). Some of the peripherally located tumor cells appear to be in the process of breaking away from the cluster. Note the nuclear hyperchromasia, multiple nucleoli, and markedly abnormal nuclear-to-cytoplasmic ratio, with only a relatively thin and markedly basophilic rim of cytoplasm (compelling evidence of malignancy).

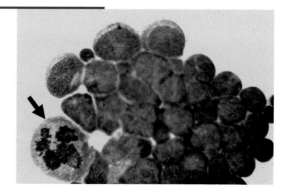

Ganglioglioma

Ganglioglioma is listed in the WHO classification as one of nine subtypes of "neuronal and mixed glioneuronal tumors." These tumors display positive immunocytochemical reactions to both neuronal and glial antigens and react with antibodies to the CD34 antigen. Ganglioglioma is usually benign (WHO grade I) but sometimes occurs in an anaplastic variant (WHO grade III). *Gangliocytoma* is a special type of ganglioglioma consisting exclusively of neoplastic ganglion cells; it can be difficult to distinguish from a neuronal hamartoma.

There are no data in the literature regarding the possible exfoliation of ganglioglioma cells into the CSF. The cytological preparations in our own two cases revealed highly malignant cells according to the standard tumor cell criteria (Figs. 5.**40**, 5.**41**). The cell nucleus is hyperchromatic, rounded, or polymorphic. The large and conspicuous nucleoli can be taken as cytological evidence of the original ganglion cell structure. The cytoplasm is strongly basophilic, and the nuclear-to-cytoplasmic ratio is significantly shifted toward the nucleus.

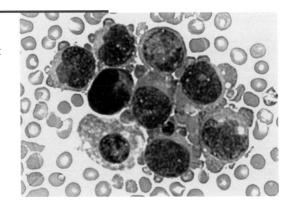

Fig. 5.**40** Cluster of tumor cells of varying degrees of viability in a patient with a ganglioglioma. The nuclei vary in size and shape large amounts of chromatin and large nucleoli, and the nuclei are partially vacuolated. Note the relatively abundant, irregular, markedly basophilic, and partially vacuolated cytoplasm. There is evidence of artifactual admixture of blood.

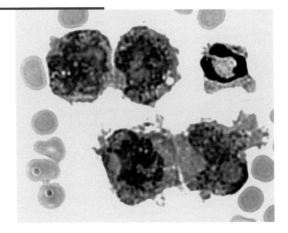

Fig. 5.**41** Tumor cells with irregularly structured nuclei and cytoplasm, and large nucleoli, in a patient with a ganglioglioma. The cytoplasm is loose, vacuolated, and basophilic, with an irregular periphery. Compare the size of these cells with that of the neighboring erythrocytes and granulocyte.

Pineal Tumors

The two main types of neuroepithelial tumor derived from the pinealocytes of the pineal body include pineocytoma (pinealocytoma, pinealoma) and pineoblastoma (pinealoblastoma). The pineal gland can also be the site of parenchymal tumors with features of both of these tumor types (pineal parenchymal tumors of intermediate differentiation).

Pineocytoma is a slowly growing, encapsulated, and often cystic tumor of WHO grade II. It consists of nests of large, clear cells interspersed with streaks of small cells resembling lymphocytes (anisomorphism). *Pineoblastoma* is a malignant tumor with marked cellular polymorphism and an elevated mitotic rate, which infiltrates the neighboring parenchyma as it grows; it is histologically similar to medulloblastoma and is assigned WHO grade IV. *Pineal parenchymal tumors* should probably be assigned a WHO grade III.

Larger pineal tumors compress or infiltrate the midbrain tectum and may compromise the cerebral aqueduct or the posterior portion of the third ventricle, causing occlusive hydrocephalus. Among the various types of pineal tumor, *pineoblastoma* is the most likely to metastasize via the CSF pathways; exfoliated cells in the CSF are sometimes seen in cases of pineocytoma, but much more commonly in cases of pineoblastoma. The cells in the CSF found in association with an *anisomorphic pinealoma* consist of small tumor cells with very little cytoplasm, resembling lymphocytes, and larger, polyploid tumor cells containing more cytoplasm and large nucleoli (Fig. 5.**44**). Polymorphic cells derived from pineocytomas vary greatly in their nuclear and cytoplasmic structure; they have a hyperchromatic nucleus, large nucleoli, and marked cytoplasmic basophilia (Fig. 5.**46**). Special reactive cell types that accompany processes in the pineal area can sometimes complicate the detection and differential diagnosis of pineal lesions, as will be shown in the case of pineal cysts (Figs. 5.**42**, 5.**43**).

It should be noted here that primary intracranial germ cell tumors also arise in the epiphysis, and cells from these tumors can exfoliate into the CSF. More will be said about this below in the section on Melanoma.

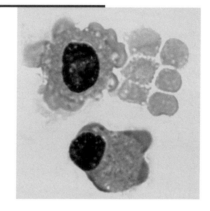

Fig. 5.**42** Reactive cells in a *pineal cyst* as an illustration of the need to differentiate such cells form tumor cells and tumor-suspect cells. In case of doubt, immunocytochemical studies are indicated for reliable differentiation.

Fig. 5.**43** Cytological preparation of CSF cells in a patient with a *pineal cyst*, revealing reactive cell types, with marked anaplasia, in a loose cluster. In contrast to the cells shown in Fig. 5.**42**, these must be considered tumor-suspect cells. They are relatively uniform and have a mainly round, but sometimes lobulated nucleus, an abnormal nuclear-to-cytoplasmic ratio in some of the cells, and a basophilic rim of cytoplasm. The adjacent erythrocytes provide an indication of the scale. Immunocytochemical tumor marker tests are indicated.

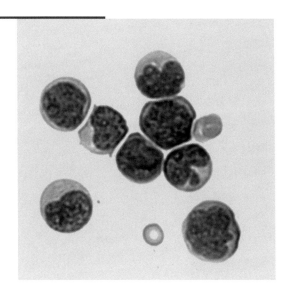

Fig. 5.**44** Anisomorphic pinealoma. Small cells containing little cytoplasm and resembling lymphocytes are seen along with a binucleated, polyploid giant tumor cell with large nucleoli and a markedly basophilic cytoplasm that has a honeycomb appearance. The overall affinity for stain is high. A few erythrocytes are also present and provide an indication of the scale.

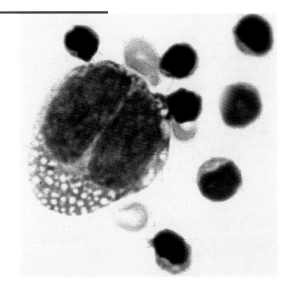

Fig. 5.**45** Small, loose tumor cell clusters in a patient with a pineocytoma. The cells have a compact nucleus of variable shape, and nucleoli; homogeneous, partly vesiculated cytoplasm; markedly increased affinity for stain; and predominant acidophilia (evidence of cell degeneration). The ring-like areas at the periphery of the cells are conceivably filled with cellular secretions. The erythrocytes indicate the scale.

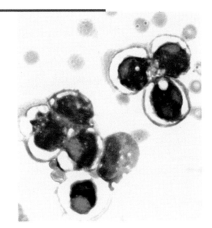

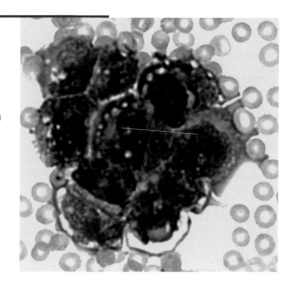

Fig. 5.**46** Tumor cell cluster with coarsely granulated, chromatin-rich nuclei, an abnormal nuclear-to-cytoplasmic ratio, and markedly basophilic, vesiculated, peripherally irregular rim of cytoplasm in a patient with a pineocytoma. Many erythrocytes are also seen, and there is abundant evidence of degeneration of multiple tumor cells.

Medulloblastoma

The current WHO classification of brain tumors assigns *medulloblastoma* grade IV and places it in the group of highly malignant *embryonal tumors* that also includes cerebral neuroblastoma, ependymoblastoma, and primitive neuroectodermal tumor (PNET) (all of these are also grade IV tumors). Medulloblastoma was previously considered a sarcomatous neoplasm of mesenchymal origin.

Grade IV medulloblastoma has a number of histopathological variants of varying prognosis: desmoplastic medulloblastoma, medullomyoblastoma, large-cell medulloblastoma, medulloblastoma with extensive nodularity, and melanotic medulloblastoma (this variant has foci of tumor cells containing melanin).

The findings of immunocytological studies have led most research groups to conclude that medulloblastoma and related types of neuroectodermal tumor arise from an *early, pluripotent neural stem cell* that normally differentiates into *both* neuronal and glial cell types. Medulloblastoma tissue, for instance, reacts both with antibodies against the neuronal antigens synaptophysin and neurofilament protein and with antibodies against the glial antigen GFAP. It does not react (or only rarely reacts) with antigens against the cytokeratins and epithelial membrane antigen (EMA).

Medulloblastoma usually arises from the roof of the fourth ventricle and grows into the lower portion of the cerebellar vermis and into both cerebellar hemispheres. It tends to *seed the meninges* and to *metastasize along the CSF pathways*, giving rise to "drop metastases," which are characteristically found among the lumbar nerve roots.

Autopsy studies of patients who died of medulloblastoma reveal metastatic disease traveling along the CSF pathways in about a third of cases. CSF examination during life reveals exfoliated tumor cells of variable size; most of these cells are smaller and relatively isomorphic (about as large as a lymphocyte or lymphoblast), but larger and multinucleated cell types may also be seen occurring singly, in small groups, or in loose clusters (Figs. 5.**47**–5.**53**). Medulloblastoma cell nuclei are hyperchromatic, rounded, often vesiculated, and interrupted by folds and invaginations. Some have a prominent nucleolus. There is usually very little cytoplasm. Depending on the degree of differentiation of the tumor, the cytoplasm may display intense basophilia, particularly in the vicinity of the cell membrane. The nuclear-to-cytoplasmic ratio is usually markedly elevated (shifted toward the nucleus). Rare polyploid cells and mitoses are seen (Figs. 5.**49**–5.**53**). In addition to the medulloblastoma cells themselves, the CSF may also display a reactive pleocytosis, which may contain eosinophilic granulocytes among other cell types.

With regard to differential diagnosis, medulloblastoma cells are sometimes difficult to distinguish from lymphoblasts or immature lymphocytes, which they resemble in their morphological and staining characteristics. When in doubt, the CSF cytologist should apply the appropriate immunocytochemical marker tests.

Retinoblastoma is a special and very rare entity. Like medulloblastoma, this *malignant retinal tumor* is said to arise from an undifferentiated precursor cell of the glial and neuronal series (an early neural stem cell); an alternative designation for it is *medulloblastoma of the retina*. We have found tumor cell clusters in the CSF of a patient with metastatic retinoblastoma (Figs. 5.**54**, 5.**55**). They consisted of isomorphic, lymphoblastlike tumor cells with one or two relatively large nucleoli, pathological mitoses, and other characteristic features of malignant neoplastic cells.

Fig. 5.**47** Tumor-suspect cells in a patient with a medulloblastoma. One cell is in the process of separating from the other. The nucleus is polyploid with large nucleoli. The nuclear constrictions indicate amitotic division. The cytoplasm is loose and basophilic with a partly irregular border. The accompanying lymphocyte provides an indication of the scale.

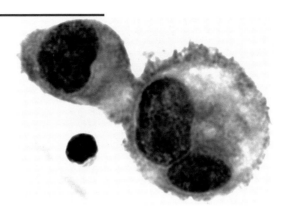

Fig. 5.**48** Atypical signet-ringlike cell with an eccentric nucleus and three other nuclei with areas of perinuclear clearing in a patient with a medulloblastoma. The cytoplasm is markedly basophilic and has a smooth periphery. These findings arouse the suspicion of abnormal differentiation, endocytogenesis, or tumor-cell cannibalism. Nearby are nuclear fragments and two degenerated monocytes.

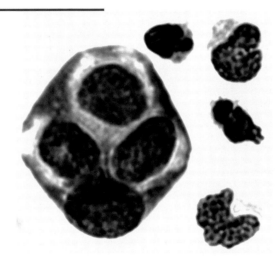

Fig. 5.**49** Tumor cells in a patient with medulloblastoma displaying variable nuclear size, nuclear-to-cytoplasmic ratio, and affinity for stain. Most of the cells have a thin rim of strongly basophilic and partially vacuolated cytoplasm. Pathological mitoses in prophase are seen (arrows). The tumor cell in the bottom right corner contains a degenerating hyperchromatic auxiliary nucleus (arrowhead).

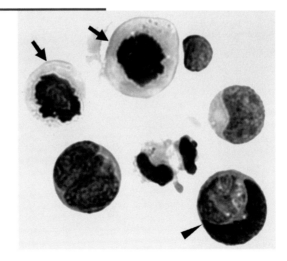

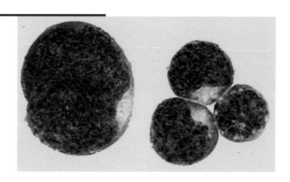

Fig. 5.**50** Isomorphic tumor cells of varying sizes, with a markedly abnormal nuclear-to-cytoplasmic ratio, in a patient with a uniform medulloblastoma. The nucleus has finely structured chromatin and nucleoli, and there is a very thin rim of basophilic cytoplasm with internal brightening. The cell on the left is a polyploid giant cell. Lymphoblasts also enter into the differential diagnosis.

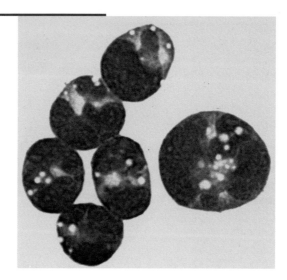

Fig. 5.**51** Tumor cells in a patient with a uniform medulloblastoma. The nucleus is polymorphic, finely granulated, and hyperchromatic and has a single nucleolus. The rim of cytoplasm is very thin in places. Vesicular inclusions are seen both in the nuclei and in the cytoplasm. The cell on the right is a polyploid giant cell.

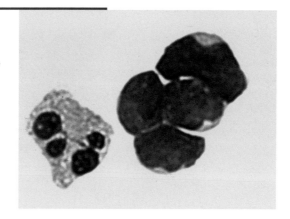

Fig. 5.**52** A relatively small, isomorphic, chromatin-rich tumor cell aggregate in a patient with a medulloblastoma. The cells have a very thin rim of basophilic cytoplasm. The cell on the left, a granulocyte, is part of the accompanying reaction (reactive pleocytosis) and provides an indication of the scale.

Fig. 5.**53** Tumor cell cluster with chromatin-rich nuclei with nucleoli, an abnormal nuclear-to-cytoplasmic ratio, and lightly basophilic cytoplasm of variable extent in a patient with a uniform medulloblastoma. Pathological mitosis in prophase (clumping of nuclear chromatin) is seen with copious, sharply demarcated, and only lightly stained cytoplasm. Lymphoblasts could conceivably enter into the differential diagnosis.

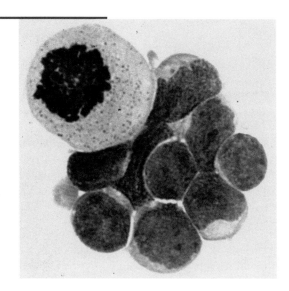

Fig. 5.**54** Cluster of tumor cells of relatively uniform morphology (neoplastic meningitis) in a patient with a retinoblastoma. The cluster is characterized by nuclei with coarsely structured chromatin and numerous nucleoli of variable size. The nuclear-to-cytoplasmic ratio is abnormal; the cytoplasm is basophilic and of variable extent. Two pathological mitoses in prophase are seen in the center of the cluster (clumping of nuclear chromatin). At the periphery, individual tumor cells are beginning to break away from the cluster. The cellular structures show evidence of degenerative change.

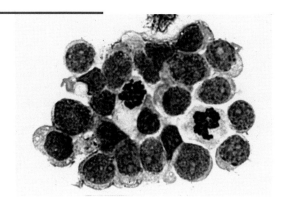

Fig. 5.**55** Cluster of nearly isomorphic tumor cells from the same patient as in Fig. 5.**54**. Features of the cells include an abnormal nuclear-to-cytoplasmic ratio; clearly visible nucleoli of variable size, and hyperchromasia. Several tumor cell fragments are also seen. The cells resemble lymphoblasts.

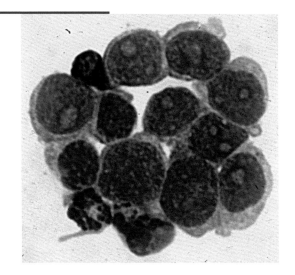

Pituitary Adenoma

The current WHO classification no longer lists pituitary adenoma as a tumor of the nervous system, but rather as an endocrine tumor. Nonetheless, we feel it is appropriate to consider pituitary adenoma in the present chapter, considering that 10–20 % of all intracranial tumors are of this type. Most pituitary adenomas are histopathologically benign (WHO grade I).

The traditional histological classification of pituitary adenomas into basophilic, eosinophilic, and chromophobic adenomas, and mixtures of these types, has fallen out of favor because of the imperfect correlation between the type and degree of staining in classic cytological preparations and the type of hormone that the tumor secretes (if any). Currently, the preferred classification is by function: the two main types of pituitary tumor are thus the *endocrine-active* tumors (approximately 60 %) and the *endocrine-inactive* tumors (the remainder). The endocrine-active tumors are further subdivided, in order of decreasing prevalence, into *prolactin-, adrenocorticotropic hormone (ACTH)-, growth hormone (GH)-, follicle-stimulating hormone/luteinizing hormone (FSH/LH)-, and thyroid-stimulating hormone*

(TSH)-secreting adenomas, though it should be noted that some tumors secrete more than one type of hormone. Tissue and serum tests relating to the hormone-secreting properties of these tumors are currently used routinely and successfully as functional methods of determining the type of pituitary adenoma that is present. *Atypical* pituitary adenoma (WHO grade II) is rare, and *anaplastic* pituitary adenoma, or *pituitary carcinoma* (WHO grade III), is very rare.

The literature contains only a few descriptions of exfoliation of pituitary adenoma cells into the CSF. References going back several decades concerning exfoliation of basophil adenoma cells can be found in Zettl et al. (2003, 2005) and Schmidt (1978, 1987), although we have reservations about the interpretation of some of the illustrations in Schmidt (1978). In the present atlas we only show, from our own case series, an example of small adenoma cells with features of cells from a tumor that was classified, by the traditional criteria, as an *eosinophilic adenoma* (i. e., a prolactinoma and/or GH-secreting adenoma) (Fig. 5.**56**). See the figure legend for further details.

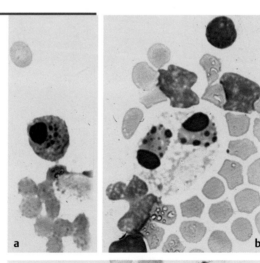

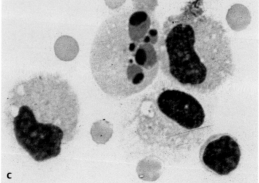

Fig. 5.**56a–c** Lightly basophilic (**a**) and eosinophilic (**b**, **c**) cells in CSF from the nose (rhinorrhea) in a patient with an eosinophilic pituitary adenoma. Small adenoma cells are seen with a compact, peripheral, chromatin-rich nucleus. The eosinophilic granules lie within an acidophilic cytoplasm with a relatively smooth border. Erythrocytes and lymphocytes (**b**, **c**) and activated monocytes (**c**) are also present and provide an indication of the scale.

Mesenchymal, Non-Meningothelial Tumors

The overall group of *tumors of the meninges* comprises the "meningothelial" tumors (i. e., meningiomas), "*mesenchymal, non-meningothelial tumors*," and "*primary melanocytic lesions*" (for the last, see Melanoma).

We have already mentioned in the first section of this chapter the lack of exfoliation of tumor cells into the CSF in most meningiomas (WHO grades I and II), and the occasional exfoliation of tumor cells in anaplastic meningiomas (WHO grade III), which are very rare. Exfoliation of tumor cells into the CSF is a much more common feature of the *mesenchymal, non-meningothelial tumors.* These neoplasms of mesenchymal origin are, however, considerably rarer than the benign meningiomas.

The group designation "mesenchymal, non-meningothelial tumors" was first used in this precise formulation in the current WHO classification (2000). This group of tumors comprises a broad spectrum of 21 entities that differ widely in their cellular differentiation and degree of malignancy. Fourteen of them were newly added to the group on histogenetic grounds in 2000, not having belonged to it in the earlier classification of 1993 (these 14 are indicated in italics): lipoma, *angiolipoma, hibernoma, liposarcoma, solitary fibrous tumors, fibrosarcoma*, malignant fibrous histiocytoma, *leiomyoma, leiomyosarcoma, rhabdomyoma*, rhabdomyosarcoma, chondroma, chondrosarcoma, osteoma, *osteosarcoma, osteochondroma, hemangioma, epithelioid hemangioendothelioma*, hemangiopericytoma, *angiosarcoma*, and *Kaposi sarcoma.*

The broad spectrum of tumors in this group reflects the enormous differentiation capacity of the *multipotent mesenchymal stem cell.* (Research on this cell type has advanced greatly over the past decade be-cause of the newly developed techniques for isolation of the mesenchymal stem cell fraction of human bone marrow.) Cells that exfoliate into the CSF from tumors of this group are correspondingly varied in shape. Any attempt to diagnose the type of tumor from the CSF cytological preparation alone would be speculative, as these cells are variable in all of the tumor cell criteria that were listed earlier in this chapter. The main question that can be answered from a May–Grünwald–Giemsa preparation is, therefore, just the simple yes-or-no question whether tumor or tumor-suspect cells are present. We think the CSF cytologist should still be permitted to follow the usage of the neurological literature and to use the term *meningeal sarcoma* (or meningeal sarcomatosis) to describe a positive finding, at least until the neuropathologist or neurooncologist has been able to make a more precise diagnosis, even though this term is not to be found in the current WHO classification. We have used this term in the figure legends in this atlas, because, besides other reasons, some of the preparations shown date back to a time when a precise diagnosis according to present criteria was not possible (Figs. 5.**57**–5.**65**).

Nonetheless, some degree of classification from the cytological preparation alone is possible for osteogenic sarcoma (Figs. 5.**67**, 5.**68**) and, to a limited extent, for malignant fibrous tumors (Fig. 5.**66**). The particular difficulty of differentiating *giant cell sarcoma* from giant cell glioblastoma, which is possible only with the use of immunocytochemical markers (vimentin, GFAP), has been mentioned in the section on Astrocytic Tumors above.

The accompanying inflammatory reactions may also be seen (Fig. 5.**60**).

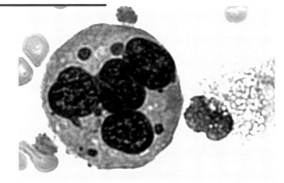

Fig. 5.**57** Tumor-suspect cell with four nuclei in a patient with meningeal sarcoma. The nuclei are isomorphic, chromatin-rich, and well demarcated, with clearly visible nucleoli. Multiple nuclear fragments (accessory nuclei?) or chromatin fragments are seen in the markedly basophilic cytoplasm, which is vacuolated in the perinuclear regions. Degenerated storage cell, erythrocytes provide an indication of the scale.

Fig. 5.**58** Clusters of possibly tumor cells in a patient with meningeal sarcoma (with evidence of mesenchymal origin). Features include marked polymorphism of nucleus and cytoplasm with markedly abnormal nuclear-to-cytoplasmic ratio; polychromasia; and a single nucleolus. The cytoplasm is partially vacuolated and has an irregular border with protuberances (pseudopodia), simulating phagocytosis and there is evidence of cell degeneration . If it is indicated for diagnostic purposes, the identity of these cells as tumor cells should be confirmed with immunocytochemical tumor marker tests. The erythrocytes indicate the scale.

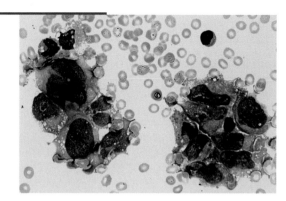

Fig. 5.**59** Relatively uniform tumor cells in a loose cluster in a patient with meningeal sarcoma. Abnormal nuclear-to-cytoplasmic ratio, nucleoli, polychromasia, and degenerative features can be seen.

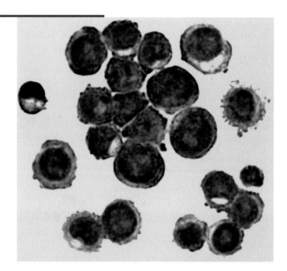

Fig. 5.**60** Meningeal sarcoma with accompanying granulocytic meningitis. Both the individual cells and the cell clusters have markedly abnormal nuclear-to-cytoplasmic ratio, marked polymorphism, polychromasia (particularly of the nucleus), and large nucleoli. The cytoplasm is strongly basophilic at the periphery and contains vacuoles. An epithelial cell (arrow) and damaged granulocytes (arrowheads) are also seen.

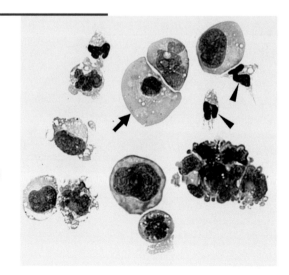

Fig. 5.**61** Loose cluster of uniform cells in a patient with meningeal sarcoma. Some of the tumor cells are connected to the cluster only by cellular bridges. The cells have a large nucleus and nucleoli, hyper- and polychromasia. The cytoplasm is strongly basophilic, finely granulated, and compact, and lighter in the perinuclear region in some cells. Pathological mitoses are seen (arrows), as well as possible expulsion of nuclei (arrowheads). In the vicinity there are nuclear fragments and erythrocytes.

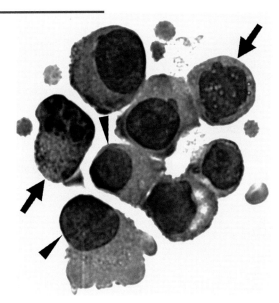

Fig. 5.**62** Tumor cell aggregate with mainly mononuclear cells (connected by cytoplasmic bridges) and one multinucleated, polyploid giant tumor cell, in a patient with meningeal sarcoma. There is marked hyper- and polychromasia. Strongly basophilic, chromatin-rich, round concretions in a rosary-bead configuration are seen at the periphery of the giant cell. Note the mitosis in prophase (arrow).

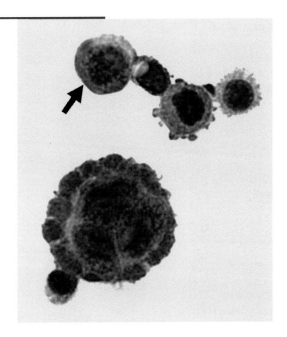

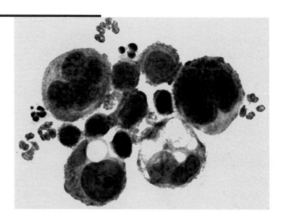

Fig. 5.**63** Mono- and multinucleated tumor cells in a loose cluster in a patient with meningeal sarcoma. The nuclei have a single nucleolus. The basophilic and acidophilic cytoplasm has vacuoles in some areas. There are strongly staining nuclear fragments in the interior of the cluster. There is reactive pleocytosis with damaged granulocytes.

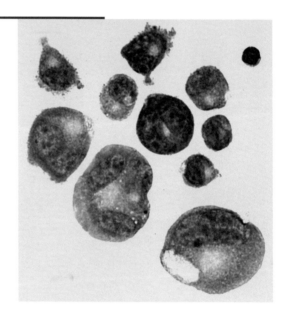

Fig. 5.**64** Tumor cells in a patient with undifferentiated meningeal sarcoma with polymorphic cells, sometimes multinucleated, with variable ploidy; numerous nucleoli; relatively large, markedly basophilic cytoplasm that is lighter in some regions, particularly in perinuclear areas. Plasmocytoma would enter into the differential diagnosis of this cytological picture.

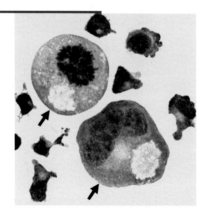

Fig. 5.**65** Polymorphic mono- and multinucleated tumor cells in a patient with undifferentiated meningeal sarcoma. The basophilic cytoplasm has bright perinuclear areas and a suggestion of glandular secretion (arrows). Mitosis in prophase is seen. Plasmocytoma would enter into the differential diagnosis of this image. Surrounding the large tumor cells are smaller tumor cells and chromatin fragments.

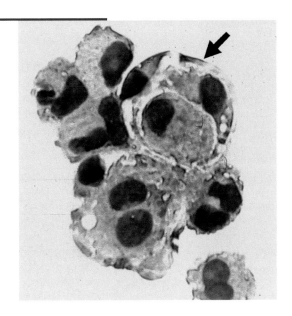

Fig. 5.**66** Cluster of mono- and bi-nucleated cells that are likely to be tumor cells in a patient with *malignant fibrous histiocytoma.* The chromatin-rich nuclei have highly variable morphology. A signet-ring form (arrow) is seen, containing viable cells (endocytogenesis? cell cannibalism?). The large, finely or coarsely granulated acidophilic cytoplasm with thickened periphery displays increased affinity for stain (pigment?). In their shape and structure, these cells closely resemble activated phagocytic cells of leptomeningeal origin.

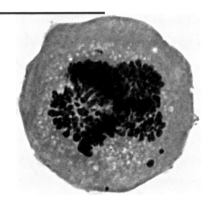

Fig. 5.**67** Polyploid giant tumor cell in mitosis (multipolar) in a patient with osteogenic sarcoma. There is relatively abundant, lightly acidophilic cytoplasm with perinuclear loosening. A few chromatin granules are also seen.

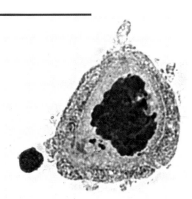

Fig. 5.**68** Polyploid giant tumor cell in mitosis in a patient with osteogenic sarcoma. Some chromatin fragments are seen. The cytoplasm is of variable appearance: lightly acidophilic in the perinuclear region, but ringlike, coarsely granulated, and basophilic at the periphery, with protuberances (pseudopodia).

Germ Cell Tumors

The WHO classification of 2000 considers *germ cell tumors* to be distinct from embryonal tumors and subdivides them into the following entities: *germinoma, embryonal carcinoma, choriocarcinoma, yolk sac tumor, teratoma* (three variants), and *mixed germ cell tumors*. Germ cell tumors can arise intracranially or metastasize to the head from the gonads; both primary and secondary intracranial germ cell tumors can spread to the leptomeninges and therefore become detectable by CSF cytological examination. The histological fine structure of an intracranial germ cell tumor and its propensity to spread to the leptomeninges are independent of whether it is primary or secondary; thus, CSF cytological examination cannot be used to determine where a germ cell tumor originated. It can, however, provide important diagnostic clues about the type of tumor that is present.

Primary intracranial germ cell tumors arise in early life from *quiescent* germ cells ("primordial germ cells") that were left behind at certain sites as undifferentiated cells during the normal process of germ cell migration through the embryo. Favored sites include the epiphysis (pineal gland and neighboring structures), pituitary gland, and hypothalamus. The factors that promote the later development of tumors from these stranded cells are still largely unknown. Germ cell tumors that arise in the fetal and perinatal periods are mainly teratomas; those that arise in later childhood, adolescence, and young adulthood include teratoma as well as germinoma (histologically identical to testicular seminoma), embryonal carcinoma, and chorionepithelioma.

Teratomas can be either mature (with well-differentiated tissues of all germinal layers) or immature (with poorly differentiated tissue, mainly of the neuroectodermal embryonal type). They often have cysts containing mucus, sebum, hair, and keratinous debris. Some of these features of teratoma tissue can also be recognized in teratoma cell clusters that appear in the CSF (see Figs. 5.**69** and 5.**70**, showing polycystic, channel-like structures). For the development of dermoid cysts from teratomas, see Chapter 6. Intracranial germinoma, like its counterpart in the gonads (seminoma), consists of relatively large cells, spaced close together, with nuclei that have very large nucleoli. Further characteristics of germinoma include the presence of giant cells in epithelium-like, loose clusters, an irregularly bordered and variably basophilic cytoplasmic structure, and a highly variable nuclear-to-cytoplasmic ratio. Cytological preparations of seminoma cells in the CSF are displayed in Figs. 5.**71** and 5.**72**.

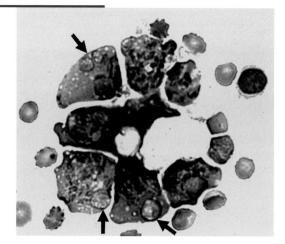

Fig.5.**69** Loose cluster of tumor cells in a patient with a teratoma that metastasized to the subarachnoid space. Nuclear morphology is highly variable, with large, occasionally compact, and chromatin-rich nuclei. Small accessory nuclei are also seen (arrows). Note the endotheliumlike arrangement of tumor cells around two centrally located, intensely hyperchromatic, cystic, channel-like structures. The mostly basophilic cytoplasm is of variable size, homogeneous or vacuolated, and has chromatin fragments. A lymphocyte and several erythrocytes indicate the scale.

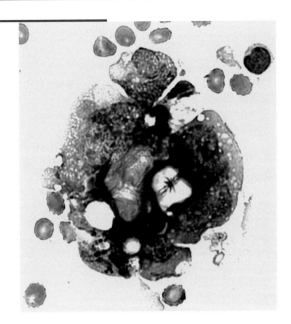

Fig. 5.**70** Tumor cell cluster in a patient with metastatic teratoma. Marked nuclear and cytoplasmic polymorphism and polychromasia are seen along with cysts of variable size—to a greater extent than in Fig. 5.**69**. The cysts are apparently partially enclosed by epidermis, which is recognizable through its high affinity for stain. The cysts apparently contain hair, other fibrous material, and a threadlike structure of some kind, with a star-shaped component. A lymphocyte and several erythrocytes provide an indication of the scale.

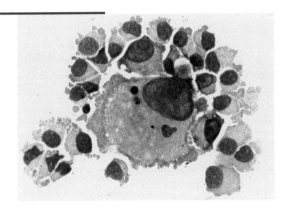

Fig. 5.**71** Loose cluster of mainly uniform-sized tumor cells with an epithelioid structure, and a single polyploid giant tumor cell, in a patient with a metastatic seminoma. Variable nuclear and cytoplasmic morphology; some of the cells have nucleoli; there are chromatin fragments in the cytoplasm of the giant cell. Irregular cytoplasmic border with a partly fringed appearance; varying degrees of basophilia in the cytoplasm.

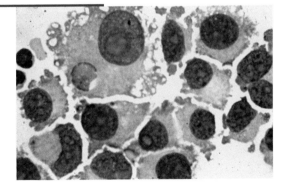

Fig. 5.**72** Loose, epitheliumlike cluster of tumor cells with a polyploid giant cell in a patient with a seminoma that metastasized to the CSF space. The giant cell cytoplasm has a hyperchromatic accessory nucleus, large to giant nucleoli, and a fringed cytoplasmic edge.

Melanoma

Melanocytic lesions arise by neoplastic degeneration of *melanocytes* or their precursor stages (*melanoblasts*). They can, therefore, be found in any tissue that possesses cells of this type, including the meninges. Melanocytic lesions in the meninges can thus be either *primary* or *metastatic*, i.e., derived from *extracranial (systemic) malignant melanoma* (direct metastasis from cutaneous or choroidal melanocytoma, or further spread from metastases in the lung, liver, etc.). The WHO classification of 2000 subdivides *primary melanocytic lesions* into *diffuse melanocytosis, melanocytoma, malignant melanoma*, and *meningeal melanomatosis*.

Conversely, malignant meningeal melanoma is a highly aggressive form of cancer that can itself give rise to distant metastases. It should be noted, however, that not every tumor that contains melanin is a melanoma. For example, a medulloblastoma, various types of glioma, a schwannoma (melanotic neurinoma), or a malignant peripheral nerve sheath tumor may contain melanin. (It is uncertain whether this is also true of anaplastic meningioma.)

Histological examination of melanocytic lesions reveals that they come in two types, *melanocytoma* and *melanoblastoma*. Tumors of the latter type grow more rapidly and their cells often exfoliate into the CSF. Cytological examination of the CSF may reveal a broad spec-

trum of *amelanotic to very strongly melanin-containing neoplastic cells,* as well as *melanophages.* These distinctive cell populations enable an unambiguous diagnosis of the disease but do *not* provide any information about its site of origin.

Melanin has a greenish-black, finely or coarsely granulated appearance in classical cytological preparations. Melanocytic tumors vary widely in the amount of melanin that they form and in the mode in which it is stored (Figs. 5.**74**–5.**80**). Melanin can also be found extracellularly (Fig. 5.**79**).

The CSF cytologist must be aware of two potential difficulties in the interpretation of May–Grünwald–Giemsa stained preparations of the CSF sediment:

1. Free melanin from dead neoplastic cells can be phagocytosed by macrophages. These macrophages, called melanophages, must not be confused with tumor cells. The cell on the left in Figure 5.**80** is an example.

2. Melanoblastoma often leads to hemorrhage into the CSF space, so that hemosiderophages may be seen alongside melanophages. Examples of these two cells are shown and contrasted in Figure 5.**81**. In case of doubt, cells of either type can be definitively identified with special stains for melanin and hemosiderin.

Fig. 5.**73** Loosely arrayed, isomorphic, mono- and multinucleated tumor cells of varying size with compact, sometimes irregular, deeply stained nuclei, in a patient with amelanotic melanoma. The cytoplasm is acidophilic and of variable density; it has a vesiculated, punched-out appearance, and its border is irregular. A pathological mitosis is seen on the left. The erythrocytes provide an indication of the scale.

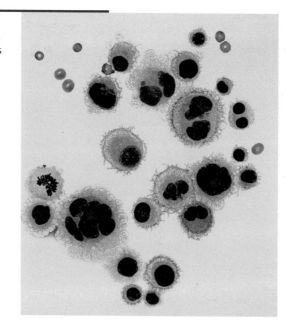

Fig. 5.**74** Loose cluster of melanotic and amelanotic, mononuclear and multinucleated, polymorphic tumor cells in a patient with a primary CNS melanoma (melanophacomatosis of Touraine type). The coarsely structured, deeply staining nuclei contain vesicles and a single nucleolus. The loose, reticulated, acidophilic cytoplasm is of variable density in the different cells. The cytoplasm in some of the cells has an irregular border and contains chromatin fragments resembling accessory nuclei. There is variable amount of melanin formation.

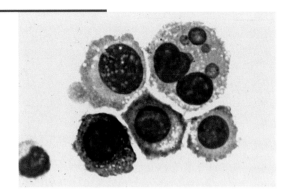

Fig. 5.**75** Loose cluster of mainly melanotic tumor cells with variable degree of melanin formation and deposition. For other characteristics see Fig. 5.**74**.

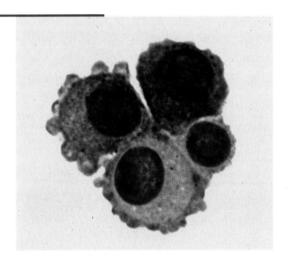

Fig. 5.**76** Isomorphic melanoma cells with fine and coarse melanin granules, alongside amelanotic, undifferentiated tumor cells.

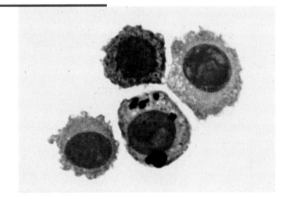

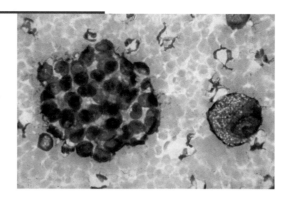

Fig.5.**77** Malignant melanoma and accompanying hemorrhage. On the left is a cluster of amelanotic tumor cells; on the right is a tumor cell containing melanin.

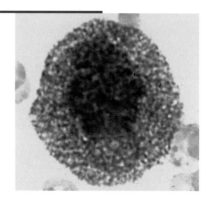

Fig. 5.**78** Mononuclear polyploid melanoblastoma cell with nuclear fragments (formation of accessory nuclei) and fine melanin granules in a patient with a primary melanoblastoma. There is evidence of accompanying hemorrhage.

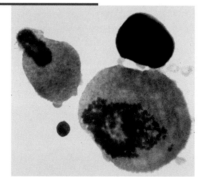

Fig. 5.**79** Tumor cells with varying amount of formation and storage of fine melanin granules. A melanoma cell expelling nuclear chromatin is seen as well as a pathological mitosis and a highly concentrated extracellular accumulation of melanin. A few erythrocytes are also seen.

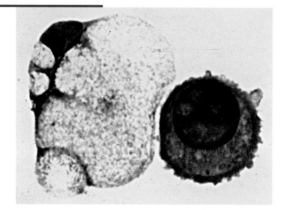

Fig. 5.**80** Signet-ring–shaped melanophage (left) and a mononuclear tumor cell in a patient with melanotic melanoblastoma.

Fig. 5.**81** Differentiation of melanin-containing melanophages from hemosiderophages (when visual differentiation is not possible, special staining techniques are indicated).

a Mononuclear melanophages in a patient with malignant melanoma, containing variably dense accumulations of fine and coarse melanin granules. Note the greenish-black coloration of the melanin granules in the May–Grünwald–Giemsa preparation.

b Hemosiderophages with two nuclei (right) and four nuclei (left) in the aftermath of a subarachnoid hemorrhage. Note the blue-black coloration of the hemosiderin granules.

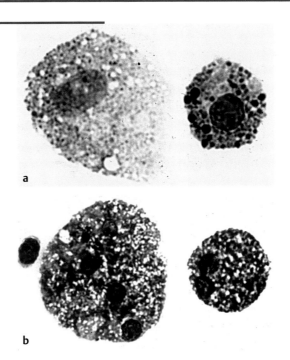

Metastases

The specialized literature has detailed information on the basic mechanisms of metastasis to the brain parenchyma (*intracerebral metastasis*) and/or the meninges (*carcinomatous meningitis*) by either the *hematogenous* or, less commonly, the *lymphatic* route. Types of tumor with a very high *rate* of metastasis include highly malignant extracranial melanoma and germ cell tumors, as well as carcinoma of the breast and lung. The types of brain metastasis that are *most commonly found* are carcinoma of the lung and breast, followed by gastrointestinal tumors and hypernephroma; tumor cells can be found in the CSF in 20–30 % of cases. The general cytological criteria for CSF tumor cells are usually clearly fulfilled by metastasis-derived cells examined in a routine May–Grünwald–Giemsa preparation.

In the spectrum of CNS metastases, the CSF cytologist can distinguish between *differentiated, undifferentiated*, and *not definitely classifiable* carcinoma cells. Differentiated carcinoma cells can be further defined in relation to the histological matrix (cell type) of the primary tumor. The CSF cytologist *cannot*, however, determine the organ of origin for any of the three types of cell.

Among all types of cerebral metastasis, CSF cells derived from *adenocarcinoma* (neoplastic glandular epithelial cells) display most clearly the histogenetic origin of the primary tumor. These cells have relatively small nuclei and a loose cytoplasm of variable architecture, containing smaller and larger vacuolar structures ("glandular" structures). These structures, which contain secretions or mucus, may become confluent and

displace the cell nucleus to the periphery, creating the so-called *signet-ring cells*. The nuclear-to-cytoplasmic ratio may be abnormal in either direction. The degree of expression of secretory activity in the cytoplasm provides a clue to the degree of differentiation of the metastatic cells. Mitoses are not very common in this cell population. The primary tumor may be, for example, an adenocarcinoma of the breast, the gastrointestinal tract, the gallbladder (Fig. 5.**100**), the female reproductive tract, or the respiratory tract (Figs. 5.**113**–5.**116**). The histological matrix of the primary tumor can also be seen relatively clearly in metastases of hypernephroma and bladder carcinoma.

In contrast, if the CSF tumor cells are of the other two types, i. e., *undifferentiated* or *not definitely classifiable*, then the histological matrix of the primary tumor can only be determined with the aid of immunocytochemical tumor marker studies. In this case, too, only the tissue type of origin of the primary tumor can be determined, rather than its precise organ of origin.

The predominantly mononuclear cells of *undifferentiated* carcinoma display a high rate of proliferation with frequent mitosis. They appear in the CSF as single cells, in groups, or in loose or compact clusters and have a markedly elevated nuclear-to-cytoplasmic ratio. The compact, hyperchromatic nuclei with coarsely structured chromatin are not always sharply delineated from the surrounding cytoplasm. The cytoplasm is usually very narrow, finely or coarsely structured, basophilic or polychromatic, and has an irregular outer border. Tumor cell cannibalism and endocytogenesis are occasionally seen. Cells of this type may be derived, for example, from undifferentiated squamous-cell carcinoma or from small-cell carcinoma of the lung (Figs. 5.**107**–5.**112** in Section 5.12.7). Examples of undifferentiated tumor cells can also be seen, of course, among the differentiated tumor cells in many of the illustrations in this chapter.

Carcinoma cells that are *not definitely classifiable* as long as the nature of the primary tumor is unknown can be seen, for example, in Figs. 5.**82**, 5.**91**, 5.**101**, 5.**107**, 5.**112**, 5.**122**, and 5.**123**. In the rest of this section on metastatic disease, we have followed the usual practice in the literature and classified the cytological preparations by the neuropathologically verified site of the primary tumor. Rather than giving further information in the text, we refer the reader to the figure legends for details.

The attentive reader will notice that we have not shown any images of CSF cells derived from extracranial tumors that very rarely metastasize into the CSF space, as we did not have the case material to do so. The type of CSF picture to be expected in such cases can be inferred from the above discussion. The prostate gland, for example, can give rise to both adenocarcinoma and squamous-cell carcinoma; thus, metastatic prostate cancer cells in the CSF might be of either of these types.

Carcinoma of the Breast

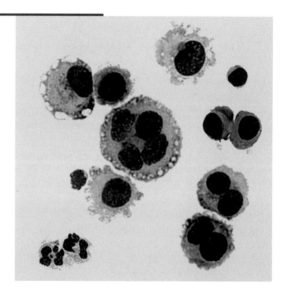

Fig. 5.**82** Mono- and multinucleated tumor cells in a patient with metastatic carcinoma of the breast. The reticulated, hyperchromatic nuclei have a single nucleolus; the cytoplasm has a relatively large, acidophilic perinuclear portion and a lightly basophilic, vacuolated peripheral portion. The granulocytes indicate the scale.

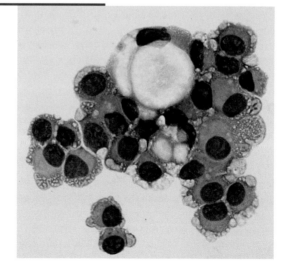

Fig. 5.**83** Relatively uniform tumor cell complex in a patient with metastatic carcinoma of the breast. Cells at the periphery of the cluster are beginning to break away. The tumor cells have a compact, hyperchromatic nucleus and a basophilic cytoplasm which, in the periphery, is vacuolated and loosened into a reticulated or cystic pattern (typical of adenocarcinoma); note the signet-ring cell with a large vacuole and a crescentic peripheral lucency (secretion?).

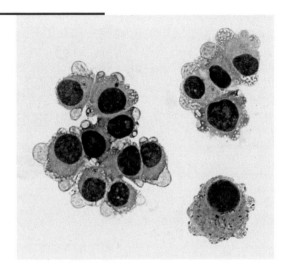

Fig. 5.**84** Features are as in Fig. 5.**83**. Also note the single large cell with acidophilic granules in the cytoplasm.

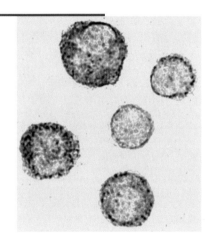

Fig. 5.**85** Tumor cells in a patient with metastatic carcinoma of the breast, *immunocytologically* characterized with the tumor marker *CK 18* (monoclonal antibody against cytokeratin subtype 18, used to identify adenocarcinoma).

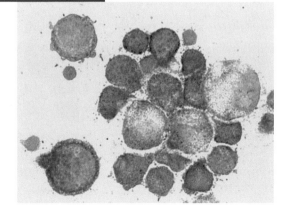

Fig. 5.**86** Tumor cells in a patient with metastatic carcinoma of the breast, *immunocytologically* characterized with the tumor marker *GCDFP 15* (monoclonal antibody against gross cystic disease fluid protein 15, used for many types of cancer, including breast cancer).

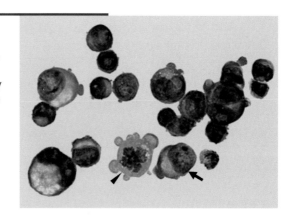

Fig. 5.**87** Loose cluster mainly containing mononuclear and binucleated cells, some of which are connected by cytoplasmic bridges, in a patient with highly aggressive metastatic carcinoma of the breast. There is marked elevation of the nuclear-to-cytoplasmic ratio, with deep staining of nuclei and cytoplasm and lighter staining in the perinuclear area (typical of adenocarcinoma). One of the tumor cells is apparently expelling its nucleus (arrow). A quadripolar mitosis (arrowhead) is seen.

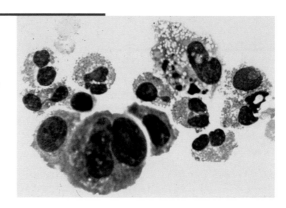

Fig. 5.**88** Mono- and binucleated tumor cells, some single and some in a cluster, in a patient with metastatic carcinoma of the breast. The large, binucleated tumor cell has elongated nuclei (early amitosis?). Many eosinophilic cells and a vacuolated storage cell with an elongated nucleus and cytoplasm contains nuclear fragments (phagocytosis?) are seen. This cytological picture illustrates a hyperergic reaction that occurred during chemotherapy, with accompanying eosinophilic meningitis.

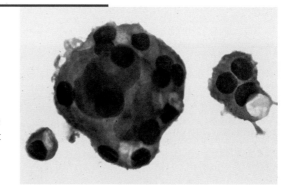

Fig. 5.**89** Suspicion of carcinomatous meningitis in a patient who developed carcinoma in the region of the surgical scar 20 years after resection and postoperative radiotherapy of a breast tumor (carcinoma). There is a cluster of cells of variable size and highly variable staining characteristics, and acidophilic or lightly basophilic cytoplasm. These cells resemble epithelial cells and they may be undergoing a transition to tumor cells?

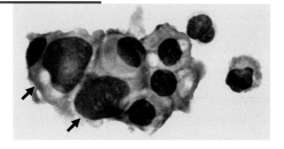

Fig. 5.**90** Cluster with cells undergoing transition to malignancy in a patient with adenocarcinoma of the breast. Two cells exhibit altered nuclear ploidy (arrows), raising a suspicion of anaplasia, whereas the remainder have relatively uniform nuclear and cytoplasmic morphology. The cytoplasm is basophilic, and partly vacuolated, with irregular borders.

Esophageal Carcinoma

Fig. 5.**91** Tumor cell clusters in a patient with metastatic carcinoma of the esophagus, with mononuclear cells in various states of viability or degeneration. The features include a large, finely granulated, chromatin-rich nucleus with high affinity for stain and a single nucleolus, and a markedly elevated nuclear-to-cytoplasmic ratio. The lower cluster contains a mitosis in prophase.

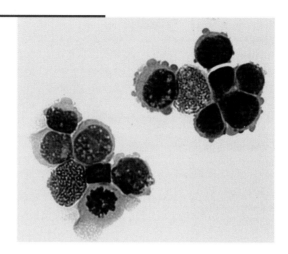

Gastric Carcinoma

Fig. 5.**92** Atypical mono- and multinucleated cells in various states of viability and degeneration in a patient with a metastatic gastric carcinoma (histologically confirmed adenocarcinoma). The nuclei are of variable size with indentations (amitosis) and numerous nucleoli. Closely apposed to the cluster is a young, viable tumor cell at an early stage of differentiation. The configuration and staining characteristics of the cytoplasm vary from cell to cell.

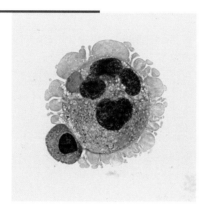

Fig. 5.**93** A number of small clusters of mononuclear tumor cells in a patient with a metastatic gastric carcinoma (histologically confirmed adenocarcinoma). The round nucleus has nucleoli, and the markedly basophilic cytoplasm shows mild perinuclear clearing. There is increased nuclear and cytoplasmic affinity for stain. Note the signet-ringlike vacuolated tumor cells and the free fragments of nuclear chromatin. The erythrocytes indicate the scale.

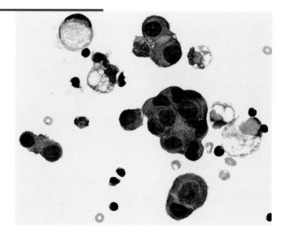

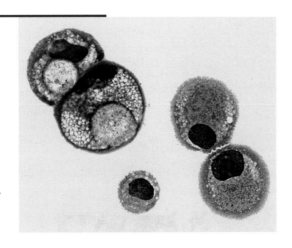

Fig. 5.**94** Tumor cells in different stages of differentiation, in the process of separating from each other, in a patient with a metastatic gastric carcinoma. The cell type is recognizable from the cell size, granulation, affinity for stain, and secretory function. The nucleus is relatively small and compact, and the copious cytoplasm of variable density has small vacuoles and some cysts. The cytoplasm is denser toward the periphery (more acidophilic centrally, more basophilic peripherally). The larger cells seem to be differentiating into signet-ring forms.

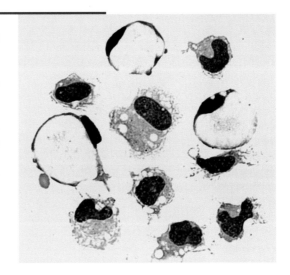

Fig.5.**95** Three typical signet-ring cells in a patient with an adenocarcinoma (metastatic gastric carcinoma), with a small, peripherally lying nucleus, basophilic cell membrane, and a large central cytoplasmic vacuole. The other cells in the vicinity cannot be unequivocally identified (tumor cells in various stages of differentiation, or else activated monocytic forms with an unusual morphology). The erythrocyte indicates the scale.

Colon Carcinoma

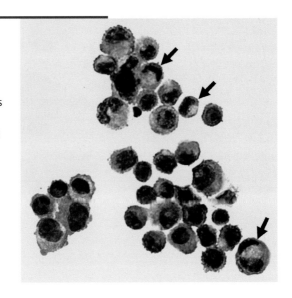

Fig. 5.**96** Loosely arranged clusters of relatively uniform tumor cells in a patient with metastatic colon carcinoma (histologically confirmed adenocarcinoma). The cells display varying stages of differentiation; different sizes of nucleus and cytoplasm, and loosening of cytoplasmic structure. Some of them are probably beginning to develop into signet-ring cells (arrows). There is marked basophilia.

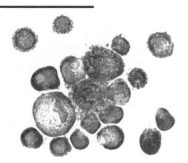

Fig. 5.**97** Tumor cells in a patient with metastatic colon carcinoma, *immunocytologically* characterized with the tumor marker *CK 18* (monoclonal antibody against cytokeratin subtype 18, used to identify adenocarcinoma).

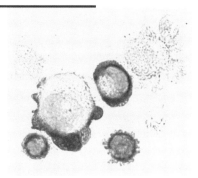

Fig. 5.**98** Tumor cells in a patient with metastatic colon carcinoma, *immunocytologically* characterized with the tumor marker *CEA* (monoclonal antibody against carcinoembryonic antigen [CEA], mainly used for suspected tumors of the colon, small intestine, and stomach).

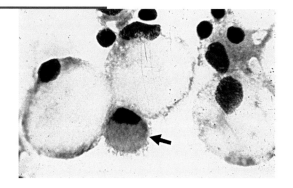

Fig. 5.**99** Cytological preparation of the CSF in a patient with metastatic colon carcinoma showing typical signet-ring cells in a cluster, with probable formation of secretions. An undifferentiated tumor cell is also seen (arrow). At the top are round, compact, hyperchromatic fragments of nuclear chromatin, some extracellular, some intracellular.

Gallbladder Carcinoma

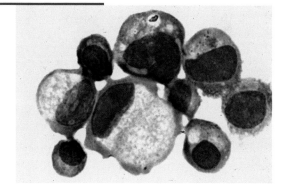

Fig. 5.**100** Loosely arranged cluster of tumor cells in a patient with metastatic adenocarcinoma of the gallbladder. The cells are interconnected by cytoplasmic bridges. Their nucleus and cytoplasm vary widely in size, shape, and staining characteristics. The cluster contains small, undifferentiated cells as well as large cells that are apparently forming secretions (signet-ring cells).

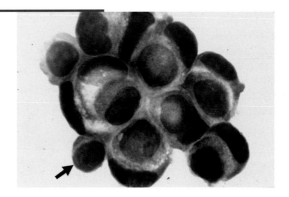

Fig. 5.**101** Cluster of relatively isomorphic tumor cells in a patient with metastatic carcinoma of the gallbladder. The cells have a compact nucleus, and some of them are in a signet-ring configuration. The partially loosened cytoplasm contains tumor cells with less strongly stained nuclei (endocytogenesis?). A small, relatively undifferentiated tumor cell (arrow) is also seen.

Cervical/Uterine Carcinoma

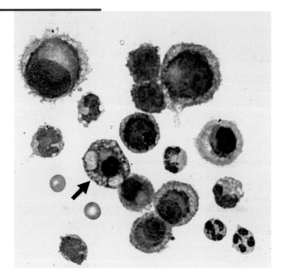

Fig. 5.**102** Tumor cells in different stages of differentiation, some of them in a loose cluster, in a patient with metastatic cervical carcinoma (histologically confirmed adenocarcinoma). The round nucleus is of variable size contains nucleoli and has increased affinity for stain. The cytoplasm is of variable morphology, compact and markedly basophilic in the perinuclear area, vacuolated to a variable extent, and less basophilic in the periphery. Early cell degeneration is seen (arrow). There is reactive pleocytosis. The granulocytes and erythrocytes indicate the scale.

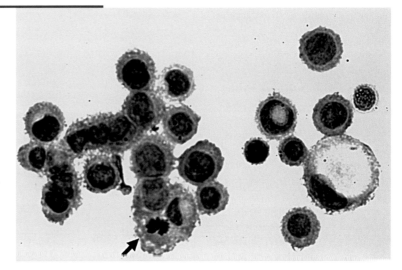

Fig. 5.**103** Tumor cells in a patient with metastatic cervical carcinoma (histologically confirmed adenocarcinoma) arranged in a loose cluster. The nuclei are round, darkly stained, and of different sizes, with large nucleoli. The basophilic cytoplasm shows varying degrees of vacuolation; there are cytoplasmic bridges between the cells. A signet-ring cell is seen on the right, and atypical mitosis (arrow) in a tumor cell with two nuclei (a main nucleus and an accessory nucleus).

Fig. 5.**104** Mono- and multinucleated tumor cells in various stages of differentiation in a patient with metastatic cervical carcinoma. Some of the cells are in a cluster. The nuclei are round with a single nucleolus. The relatively copious cytoplasm has a markedly loosened internal structure, particularly in the irregular peripheral regions, with homogeneous and finely granulated acidophilia. Atypical mitosis with clumping of the chromosomes (arrow).

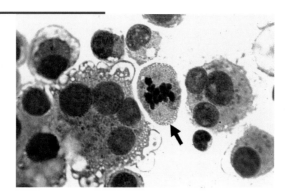

Fig. 5.**105** Mostly mononuclear, highly polyploid tumor cells in a patient with adenocarcinoma of the uterus. Some of the tumor cells are still in a cluster. The nuclei have large nucleoli. The cytoplasm is of variable size and markedly loosened, with evidence of secretory function and an indication of the tumor matrix. There is a small, not yet differentiated tumor cell (arrow). Mitosis in anaphase is seen (upper right corner).

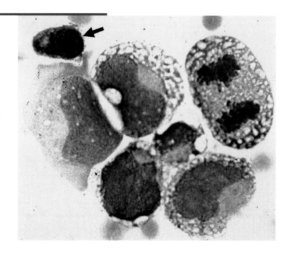

Fig. 5.**106** Mononuclear, polyploid tumor cells at different stages of differentiation, some of them connected to other tumor cells, in a patient with adenocarcinoma of the uterus. The cytoplasm is markedly reticulated or vacuolated and lightly basophilic. Nucleoli are large, and pathological mitoses in metaphase (arrow) and anaphase can be seen. The erythrocytes provide an indication of the scale.

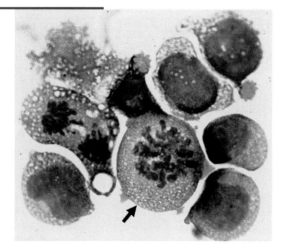

Carcinoma of the Respiratory Tract

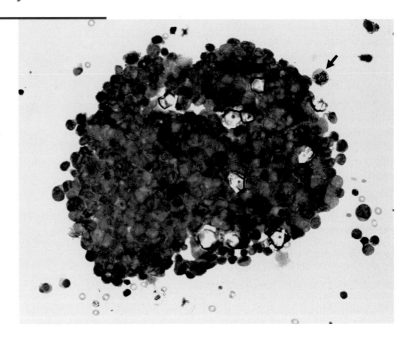

Fig. 5.**107** An extremely large, multi-layered cluster of heavily staining tumor cells in a patient with an undifferentiated bronchial carcinoma. Cells at the periphery are breaking away from the cluster. The nuclear-to-cytoplasmic ratio is abnormal. Pathological mitosis is seen (arrow). The erythrocytes provide an indication of the scale.

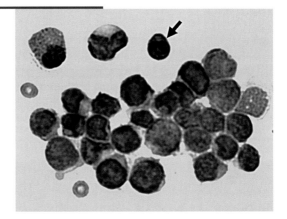

Fig. 5.**108** Uniform tumor cells in a patient with small-cell carcinoma of the lung. Large cells with markedly abnormal nuclear-to-cytoplasmic ratio and many nucleoli. There are cytoplasmic bridges between the cells and a single undifferentiated cell (arrow) is seen. The erythrocytes provide an indication of the scale.

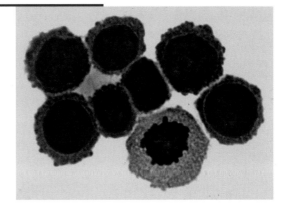

Fig. 5.**109** Loose cluster of tumor cells in a patient with highly malignant small-cell carcinoma of the lung, with markedly abnormal nuclear-to-cytoplasmic ratio; blurred demarcation, in places, of the nucleus from the surrounding cytoplasm; heavy staining; and irregular cell border. Pathological mitosis in prophase is seen.

Fig. 5.**110** Uniform tumor cells in a patient with an undifferentiated bronchial carcinoma, with abnormal nuclear-to-cytoplasmic ratio and multiple nucleoli. The strongly acidophilic cytoplasm has a basophilic periphery. Possible endocytogenesis is occurring in the signet-ring–shaped tumor cell (arrow). The granulocyte provides an indication of the scale.

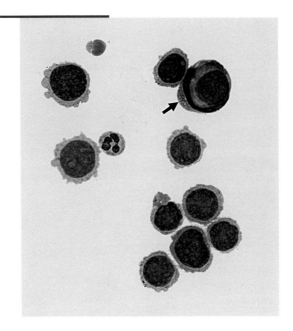

Fig. 5.**111** Loose cluster of relatively uniform tumor cells in a patient with small-cell carcinoma of the lung, with markedly abnormal nuclear-to-cytoplasmic ratio. The cells have only a thin rim of cytoplasm, with variably intense basophilic staining. In the center of the figure is a pathological mitosis (prophase, early metaphase). The few erythrocytes provide an indication of the scale.

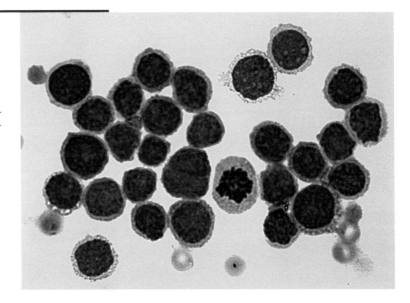

Fig. 5.**112** Tumor cells of variable size in the process of breaking away from the loose cluster in a patient with undifferentiated bronchial carcinoma. A polyploid giant tumor cell is seen (early amitosis?), as well as two smaller tumor cells with irregular cell borders. Another adjacent tumor cell is undergoing apoptosis. Many nucleoli in the viable cells.

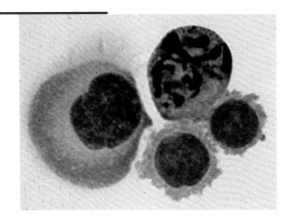

Fig. 5.**113** Tumor cells of varying size in a patient with a histologically confirmed adenocarcinoma of the lung (the CSF cell count was normal!). The nucleus is rounded, with a single nucleolus. The relatively abundant, finely structured, acidophilic cytoplasm has a smooth or finely textured border. Vacuoles and secretory granules within the cytoplasm indicate secretory function and thus point to the cell type of origin.

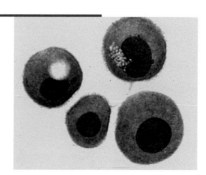

Fig. 5.**114** Pairs of tumor cells with an abnormal nuclear-to-cytoplasmic ratio in a patient with adenocarcinoma of the lung. The compact, chromaffin nucleus has a single nucleolus (the CSF cell count was normal!). The basophilic cytoplasm contains vacuoles between the nucleus (secretion?) and irregular border.

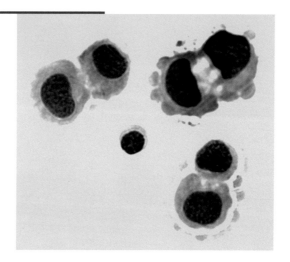

Fig. 5.**115** Specimen from a patient with a histologically confirmed adenocarcinoma of the lung: uniform tumor cells with a compact, centrally or peripherally located nucleus and relatively abundant cytoplasm with variable degrees of vacuolation; polychromasia; no evident abnormality of the nuclear-to-cytoplasmic ratio (indicates a low level of differentiation). The tumor cell at the bottom is beginning to degenerate and seems to be expelling its nucleus.

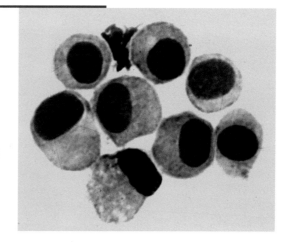

Fig. 5.**116** Mono- and multinucleated tumor cells of variable size and shape in a patient with adenocarcinoma of the lung. The relatively compact, hyperchromatic nuclei are peripherally or centrally located. The large or smaller amount of cytoplasm has pronounced, ringlike basophilia at the periphery. The cell border is either smooth or irregular; the crownlike cytoplasmic protuberances indicate an undifferentiated tumor cell. The loose cytoplasm with vacuolation and low affinity for stain indicates secretion and thus provides a clue to the histogenesis of the primary tumor.

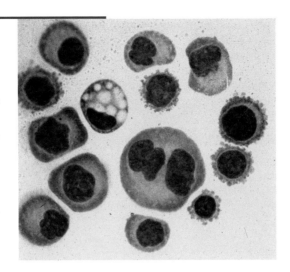

Hypernephroma

Fig. 5.**117** Single, compact tumor cell in a patient with a hypernephroma. The tumor cell has a chromatin-rich nucleus and a giant nucleolus, and a copious, finely granulated cytoplasm with smooth border. There is accompanying hemorrhage. Erythrocytes have formed a rosettelike array around the tumor cell and are linked to one another by cytoplasmic bridges (chemotaxis, adhesion phenomena).

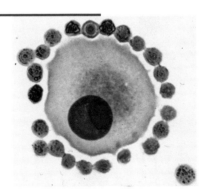

Fig. 5.**118** CSF cytological preparation in a patient with hypernephroma. The two tumor cells at the top of the figure display a "foamy" periphery and a more tightly organized, finely granulated cytoplasm in the perinuclear area, and a compact, hyperchromatic nucleus with nucleoli. There is evidence of accompanying hemorrhage with rosettelike arrangement of erythrocytes around the tumor cells. The erythro-/hemosiderophage at the bottom of the figure is evidence of an earlier accompanying hemorrhage into the subarachnoid space.

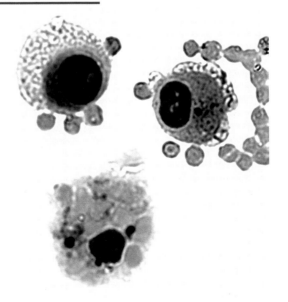

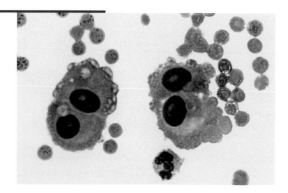

Fig. 5.**119** Binucleated tumor cells in the process of separation in a patient with hypernephroma. The compact, hyperchromatic nuclei have large nucleoli. The cytoplasm contains turquoise-colored deposits of an unknown nature; it is vacuolated is places and has prominent protuberances.

Bladder Carcinoma

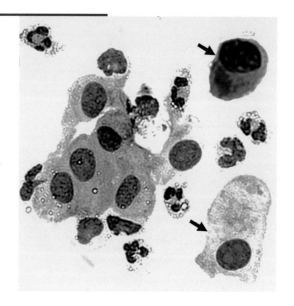

Fig. 5.**120** Mononuclear, epithelioid tumor-suspect cells in varying stages of differentiation, some of which are arranged in a cluster, in a patient with bladder carcinoma that has metastasized to the CSF space. Cylindrical epithelioid cells are seen (arrow). The copious acidophilic cytoplasm sometimes has a light basophilic tinge. There is accompanying granulocytic pleocytosis (the granulocytes provide an indication of the scale).

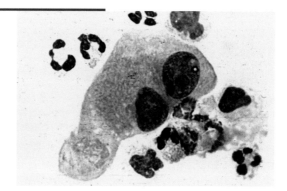

Fig. 5.**121** Binucleated, cylindrical, epithelioid tumor-suspect cell reminiscent of vesical epithelium in a patient with metastatic carcinoma of the bladder, with large nuclei and nucleoli, and abundant, finely granulated, partly acidophilic and partly basophilic cytoplasm. Reactive pleocytosis is seen.

Ethmoidal Carcinoma

Fig. 5.**122** Tumor cell clusters showing signs of mild degeneration (the CSF arrived in the laboratory 3 hours after lumbar puncture) in a patient with metastatic ethmoidal carcinoma (infiltration of the skull base). The cells show variable nuclear morphology and an abnormal nuclear-to-cytoplasmic ratio. The cytoplasm displays irregular borders, intercellular bridge formation, and partly basophilic, partly acidophilic staining (the bubbles are artifacts of preparation).

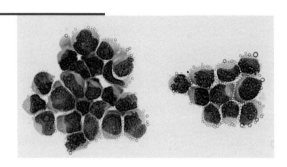

Fig. 5.**123** Loose cluster of uniform tumor cells in a patient with metastatic ethmoidal carcinoma, probably due to local infiltration of the tumor into the CSF space, with pachy- and leptomeningeal disease. The cells have a compact, vacuolated, chromaffin-rich nucleus and likewise vacuolated cytoplasm. Mitosis in prophase is seen.

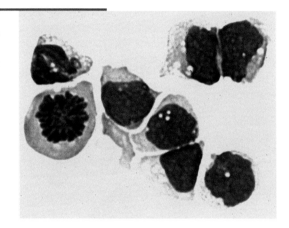

Malignant Lymphoma and Plasmacytoma

The group of tumors designated "*lymphoma and hematopoietic tumors*" in the WHO classification of 2000 is subdivided into malignant *lymphoma, plasmacytoma*, and *granulocytic sarcoma* (*chloroma*) (Radner *et al.* 2002). The further classification of lymphomas is described in the new "WHO classification of lymphomas, 2000" (Stein 2000). We have used the older Kiel classification in some of the figure legends in this section.

Malignant lymphoma manifests itself in the CNS either as *primary malignant CNS lymphoma* or as *metastasis of extracerebral lymphoma* (*generalized malignant lymphoma with isolated CNS infiltrates*). More than 90 % of all cases are *B cell lymphoma* and are characterized by *monoclonality*, as can be demonstrated by *light-chain restriction.*

Primary and metastatic B cell lymphomas are histologically identical. The CSF cytologist, therefore, has no way of determining the site of origin of B cell lymphoma cells that may be seen in the CSF sediment (lymphomatous meningitis). Metastatic CNS lymphoma does, however, tend to shed cells into the CSF more commonly, and in greater number, than primary CNS lymphoma. In some cases of primary CNS lymphoma, tumor cells do not appear in the CSF at first, but are seen later, when the tumor recurs.

Lymphoma cells in the CSF sediment, when stained with the May–Grünwald–Giemsa technique, display features of *blast precursor stages* that do not permit the cytologist to distinguish between the subgroups of malignant lymphoma, although a relative degree of polymorphism of nuclear and cytoplasmic structure can be seen, along with finely nuanced variations in the uptake of stain (Figs. 5.**124**–5.**137**). Most cells have an isomorphic appearance, with a hyperchromatic, round, usually infolded nucleus, whereas others with a conspicuously lobulated nucleus can also be seen (Figs. 5.**124**, 5.**126**, 5.**129**–5.**131**). The nucleus may contain several nucleoli, and the nuclear-to-cytoplasmic ratio is markedly elevated. The relatively thin rim of cytoplasm is usually strongly basophilic, with clearly visible Golgi zones.

The distinction between B and T cell lymphoma can only be made immunocytologically with the aid of appropriate antibody panels (see Wick in Zettl *et al.* 2003, 2005). This is usually not an issue for the CSF cytologist, because the type of lymphoma that is present has most often already been determined from other tissues. The question usually asked is simply whether lymphomatous meningitis is present, and this can be adequately answered from the classical cytological preparation alone. An immunocytochemical differentiation of the CSF preparation might be needed in cases with a low blast fraction and possibly confounding cell types, such as normal lymphoblasts, leukemia cells, or activated lymphocytes, or in primary CNS lymphoma, where no extracranial tissue is available for analysis.

Hodgkin disease arises by neoplastic transformation of B cells, mainly in the area of the neck, possibly induced by a virus (whose identity remains unknown).

We found lymphomatous meningitis in one patient with Hodgkin disease. The cytological preparation is shown in Fig. 5.**136** and described in the figure legend.

The *plasmocytomas*, or *plasmocytic neoplasms*, are subdivided into *extramedullary solitary plasmocytoma, solitary plasmocytoma of bone, the multifocal form of multiple myeloma, multiple myeloma* (*myelomatosis*), and *plasmablastic sarcoma*. All of these entities are due to *monoclonal proliferation of plasma cells and their precursor forms* (*B cell neoplasia with terminal differentiation*). Cytological preparations of neoplastic plasma cells that have infiltrated the meninges and migrated into the CSF are shown in Fig. 5.**138**. The cells are of highly variable size, but nonetheless fairly isomorphic. They are frequently multinucleated and display characteristic nuclear and cytoplasmic features, including a perinuclear Golgi zone, poly- and hyperchromasia of the nucleus, and strong basophilia of the cytoplasm. These features are all seen to a greater or lesser extent depending on the degree of differentiation and malignancy of the neoplasm.

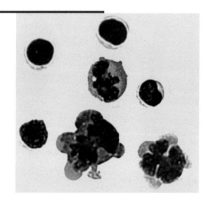

Fig. 5.**124** Typical cytological findings in lymphoma: small cells with a round nucleus and little cytoplasm; cellular fragments; larger cells with a conspicuously lobulated nucleus and basophilic cytoplasm. Clinical diagnosis: *primary B cell lymphoma.*

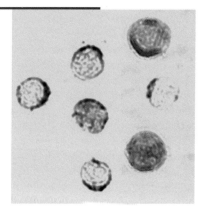

Fig. 5.**125** Lymphoma cells from the same patient as in Fig. 5.**124** with immunocytochemical staining for the *CD 20* antigen (a marker of B cells).

Fig. 5.**126** Cytological findings in centrocytic lymphoma: lymphoma cells with a round, chromatin-rich nucleus, as well as characteristically lobulated nuclear structures with vacuolation and a single nucleolus. The cytoplasm also displays vacuolar loosening and is markedly basophilic at its periphery. A few lipophages and erythrocytes are also seen.

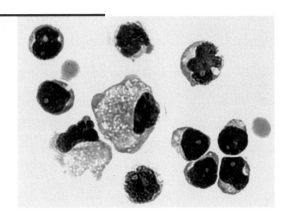

Fig. 5.**127** Cytological findings in highly malignant *primary B cell lymphoma* with marked abnormality of the nuclear-to-cytoplasmic ratio. The round or lobulated chromatin-rich nucleus is of variable size, with indentations and multiple nucleoli. There is a very thin, often barely recognizable rim of intensely basophilic cytoplasm, sometimes with an irregular border.

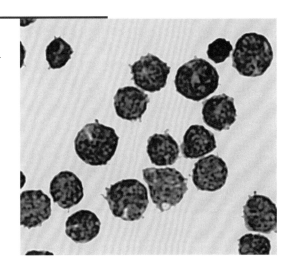

Fig. 5.**128** An illustration of variable shifting of the nuclear-to-cytoplasmic ratio; note also the nuclear and cytoplasmic hyperchromasia in this patient with *B cell lymphoma.*

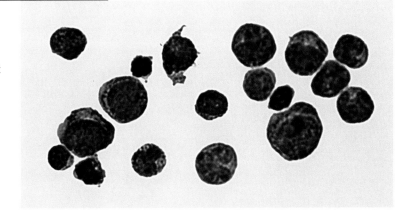

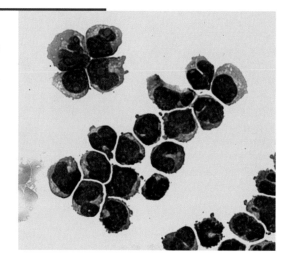

Fig. 5.**129** Typical lymphoma cells in *non-Hodgkin lymphoma,* some of which are in groups or loose clusters. The chromatin-rich, lobulated or round nucleus has a single nucleolus. the variably basophilic cytoplasm has smooth or irregular borders.

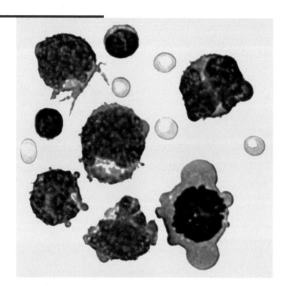

Fig. 5.**130** Typical large and small lymphoma cells in a patient with *non-Hodgkin lymphoma.* Erythrocytes indicate the scale. A mitosis in prophase is seen in the bottom right of the figure.

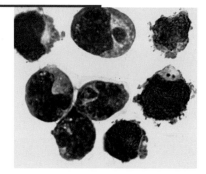

Fig. 5.**131** "Pure culture" of lymphoma cells with typical nuclear and cytoplasmic morphology, as well as poly- and hyperchromasia, in a patient with *non-Hodgkin lymphoma.*

Fig. 5.**132** Lymphoma cells of variable ploidy in a patient with *Burkitt lymphoma:* the chromatin-rich nucleus is round, lobulated, or indented, with a reticular structure and a single nucleolus. There is a thin, strongly basophilic rim of cytoplasm (markedly abnormal nuclear-to-cytoplasmic ratio).

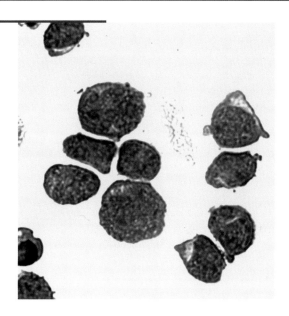

Fig. 5.**133** Lymphoma cells in "pure culture" in a patient with *Burkitt lymphoma;* the cells resemble those in Fig. 5.**132**. A pathological mitosis in anaphase (arrow) and several apoptotic cells in different stages of degeneration, e.g., vacuolation, nuclear fragmentation, are seen.

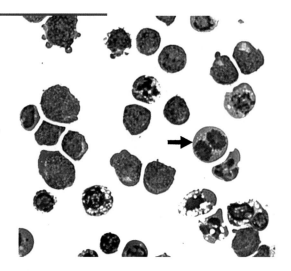

Fig. 5.**134** Neoplastic cells of variable sizes and ploidy in a patient with *primary immunoblastic malignant lymphoma of the CNS* with chromatin-rich nucleus and deeply staining cytoplasm. Note the mitosis in anaphase (top left) and quadripolar mitosis (bottom right).

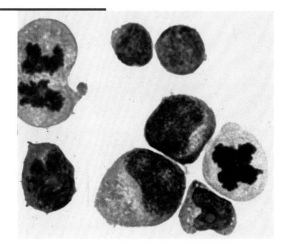

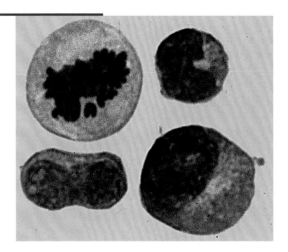

Fig. 5.**135** Neoplastic cells of different sizes and a nucleolated nucleus in a patient with *immunoblastic malignant lymphoma.* The nucleus and cytoplasm are heavily stained. At the top left is a pathological mitosis in metaphase, with breaking-off and clumping of chromosomal material; the cell directly below is undergoing amitotic nuclear division and early cell division.

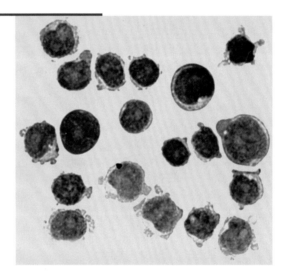

Fig. 5.**136** Lymphomatous meningitis in *Hodgkin disease:* relatively isomorphic cells in different stages of activation, with a markedly abnormal nuclear-to-cytoplasmic ratio. Unlike the neoplastic cells in other types of lymphoma, most of these cells have a round nucleus; lobulated and indented nuclei are much rarer. There are relatively large nucleoli.

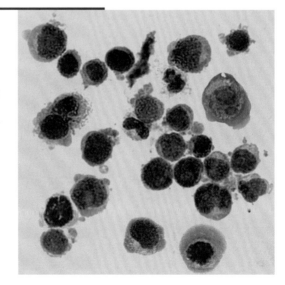

Fig. 5.**137** Clinical diagnosis: neoplastic meningitis accompanying probable *lymphoblastic malignant lymphoma* (earlier designated as lymphosarcoma). The figure shows cells of different shapes, some of them alone and others in a loose cluster. The nuclear-to-cytoplasmic ratio is abnormal and the cells have varying affinity for stain depending on the degree of differentiation.

Fig. 5.**138** CSF cytological preparation in *plasmacytoma*: various types of mono- and multinucleated neoplastic plasma cells.

a Cells of relatively typical morphology: round nuclei, mainly peripherally located, with nucleoli, perinuclear clearing, and strongly basophilic cytoplasm.

b Mono- and multinucleated neoplastic plasma cells of varying degrees of maturity: spherical clumping of nuclear chromatin (in some cells), perinuclear clearing, indistinct nuclear-cytoplasmic borders, and markedly basophilic cytoplasm with increased affinity for stain.

c Mono- and multinucleated neoplastic plasma cells of varying degrees of maturity: mostly small cells with a few large ones with formation of cell aggregates.

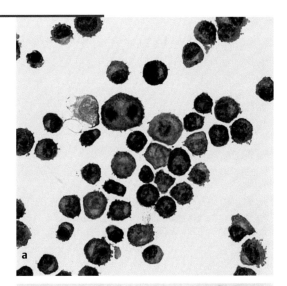

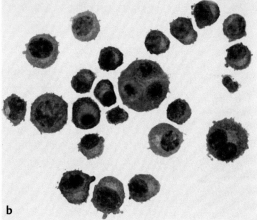

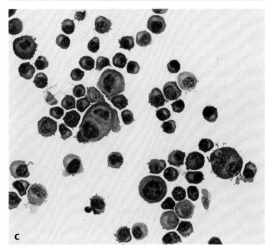

Leukemia

The conventional *FAB (French-American-British) classification* of the leukemias subdivides them into *acute lymphatic leukemia (ALL), acute myelogenous leukemia (AML)*, and the corresponding *chronic forms (chronic lymphatic leukemia [CLL], chronic myeloid leukemia [CML])*.

The reader is referred to the specialized literature in hematology and oncology for detailed discussions of the etiology and pathogenesis of these *malignant lympho- and myeloproliferative disorders*. Their *differential diagnosis* is carried out with the classical methods of cytomorphology, histology, and cytochemistry and is complemented by multiparametric immune phenotyping, fluorescence *in situ* hybridization (FISH), and the polymerase chain reaction (PCR). From the current state of research in the field, it seems clear that the classification of the leukemias will soon be further improved by gene expression analysis through *microarray technology*, so that more specific treatments can be given.

The differential diagnosis of leukemia is based on the examination of specimens of *blood and bone marrow* and is therefore the primary responsibility of the *specialist hematology laboratory*. The diagnosis has usually already been established, and the cell type determined, before the first lumbar puncture is performed. The CSF cytologist will already have the FAB diagnosis at hand when he or she is required to determine whether *leukemic meningitis* is present. The analysis of the sample by the CSF cytologist can therefore be limited to a determination of the cell count, evaluation of the classically stained sediment, and, if there are enough cells, a flow cytometric analysis (cf. Chapter 1, Diagnostic Use of Flow Cytometry in CSF Cytological Examination).

This can be to the CSF cytologist's advantage, because malignant leukemic blast forms are morphologically so similar to normal hematopoietic blast precursor cells that they may be difficult or impossible to distinguish from them in a May–Grünwald–Giemsa cytological preparation. Such cases of doubt, and certain other ones (see below), will rarely give rise to the need for the CSF cytologist, too, to resort to cytochemical or immunocytochemical differentiation techniques, using the appropriate antibody panels (see Chapter 1, Diagnostic Use of Immunocytological Phenotyping Techniques in CSF Cytology and further information in Wick's chapter in Zettl *et al.* 2003, 2005).

ALL, according to the FAB classification, is further subdivided into the *subtypes ALL-L1, ALL-L2, and ALL-L3*. In these three entities, the lymphoblasts found in the blood and bone marrow differ from one another *morphologically* in terms of cell size, nuclear-to-cytoplasmic ratio, presence of nucleoli, and regularity of nuclear and cellular shape, and are *cytochemically* char-

acterized by their patterns of coarsely granular *PAS-positive* intracellular deposits, *negative* peroxidase reaction, and *negative or, at most, weakly positive* nonspecific esterase reaction. The subtype has usually already been determined by the time of lumbar puncture; thus, in ALL, the CSF cytologist is usually asked only whether leukemic meningitis is present and is *not* required to subclassify any leukemia cells that may be found.

CSF tumor cells in ALL appear relatively isomorphic in a classical cytological preparation, though the individual blasts are often polymorphic (Figs. 5.**139**–5.**143**). There may be polyploid blasts with barely visible cytoplasm, pathological mitoses (sometimes multipolar), and degenerative forms (Figs. 5.**141**–5.**143**). The cells' affinity for stain depends on their degree of maturation and malignancy. Further lumbar punctures for the monitoring of treatment with intrathecally administered cytostatic agents may yield macrophages containing phagocytosed blasts and chromatin fragments, as well as highly polyploid giant cells, degenerative forms, and other reactive cell types (Fig. 5.**144**).

In *CLL*, the cytological features of malignancy are less pronounced. Often, one sees only a poorly differentiated lymphocytic cell picture, with barely recognizable small blasts containing very little cytoplasm.

ALL cells are most likely to be *confused* with activated inflammatory lymphocytic cells, whereas CLL cells can be confused with these or even with normal lymphocytes, resulting in an incorrect diagnosis of viral meningitis. Lymphoblasts occasionally need to be distinguished from tumor cells of other types (see Figs. 5.**9**, 5.**28**, 5.**50**, 5.**51**, 5.**53**, 5.**55**, 5.**110**, 5.**111**).

Cytochemical and immunocytochemical criteria are likewise the basis of the FAB classification's subdivision of *AML* into *three blast types* and *eight subgroups* (see Thomas 1998 and the specialized literature). Here, too, the CSF cytologist is usually asked only whether leukemic meningitis is present, i.e., whether blasts of the *myeloid* series appear in the CSF, without being required to subclassify the disease any further. The classical cell preparation, however, may enable not just the recognition of AML cells, but also a partial differentiation of immature cell types, so that the CSF cytologist can sometimes provide more specific diagnostic information: the malignant cytological features are more pronounced in myelo- and monoblasts, as well as in transitional forms displaying partial maturation into granulo- and monocytes (Fig. 5.**146**–5.**151**). A few mitoses can be seen (Fig. 5.**147**). For further details, see the figure legends.

There is usually no difficulty in distinguishing AML cells from the lymphocytic precursors of ALL in the classical cytological preparation. Sometimes, however, blast precursors of the myeloid series can be hard to tell apart from lymphoma cells (compare Figs. 5.**146**, 5.**147** with Figs. 5.**129**, 5.**132**).

In *CML*, the *peripheral blood smear* reveals all of the maturation stages of granulopoiesis, with only mild accentuation of metamyelocytes and neutrophilic granulocytes. In general, the cellular morphology is mostly normal. Eosinophilic and basophilic granulocytes are present in elevated numbers; a basophilic fraction above 20 % indicates an incipient blast phase. It is useful for the CSF cytologist if the physician sending in the CSF specimen for study provides information of this type. Depending on the phase of the disease, the CSF, too, may be found to contain elevated amounts of basophilic and eosinophilic granulocytes in addition to the myeloblasts and promyelocytes.

In *leukemia*, just as in malignant lymphoma and plasmacytoma, classical cytological examination of the CSF plays a very important role in identifying neoplastic cells in the CSF (initial manifestation and recurrences), and therefore also in determining the course of *treatment*. Particularly in leukemia, when the CSF findings are positive, a course of intrathecal chemotherapy with an appropriate agent can have an impressive, beneficial result. Blasts in the CSF may be markedly reduced in number, or even totally eliminated, in a matter of days.

As a further illustration of the extraordinary variety of malignant leukemic blast forms in leukemic meningitis, Figure **5.152** shows the morphological differences between blasts in the CSF, bone marrow, and blood of a *single patient* with *chloroma* (a special type of AML, also known as myelosarcoma).

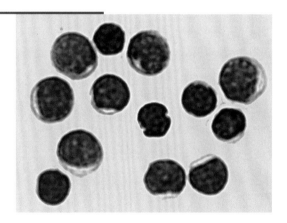

Fig. 5.**139** Blasts in leukemic meningitis due to ALL: variable amount of cytoplasm, and varying affinity for stain.

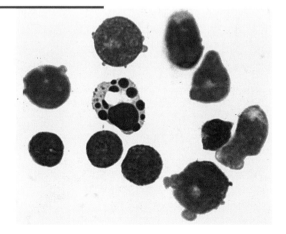

Fig. 5.**140** ALL: marked abnormality of the nuclear-to-cytoplasmic ratio; deeply staining nucleus and cytoplasm; cytoplasmic protuberances. The overall picture indicates a high degree of malignancy (see also Figs. 5.**139** and 5.**141**). There is a degenerated cell in the center of the figure (apoptosis).

Fig. 5.**141** Variable blast forms with relatively large cytoplasm and a multi-polar mitosis in a patient with ALL.

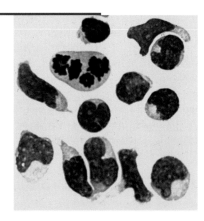

Fig. 5.**142** ALL: macroblast in the center, and above it, a mitosis in prophase or early metaphase.

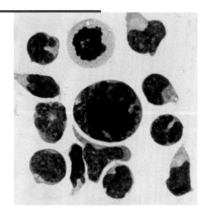

Fig. 5.**143** Lymphoblasts with nuclei of highly varied structure, some of them in a clover-leaf configuration in the CSF of a patient with ALL. The cells have only a narrow, lightly basophilic rim of cytoplasm.

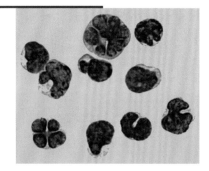

Fig. 5.**144** Leukemic meningitis in a patient with ALL, displaying different types of reactive cell induced by *treatment* involving intrathecal administration of cytostatic agents.

a Lymphoblasts and an erythrophage containing mainly digested erythrocytes—an indication of accompanying hemorrhage (due to prior lumbar puncture?).

b Highly malignant lymphoblasts and a macrophage with cytoplasmic protuberances and phagocytosed nuclear chromatin from lymphoblasts.

c Leukophage with phagocytosed cellular and nuclear fragments of blast cells damaged by the treatment, surrounded by three intact lymphoblasts.

d Macrophage containing a nearly intact lymphoblast and other blast fragments, in the process of phagocytosing three cells or cell fragments. A lymphoblast is seen in the bottom left corner.

e Macrophage containing relatively intact blasts, vacuoles, and a chromatin fragment, surrounded by lymphoblasts with abundant cytoplasm.

f Two macrophages (possibly of endothelial origin) containing phagocytosed blasts and a chromatin fragment. Around them are many lymphoblasts in various states of activation.

g Highly polyploid giant cell in leukemic meningitis, with a loosely structured nucleus and copious, partially vacuolated, finely granulated cytoplasm, which is basophilic at the periphery. Next to it are two adjacent lymphoblasts; erythrocytes are shown for scale.

h Apoptotic cell with marked clumping of chromatin, hyperchromasia and degeneration of the nucleus, and vacuolation of the cytoplasm. Adjacent to it are several intact lymphoblasts.

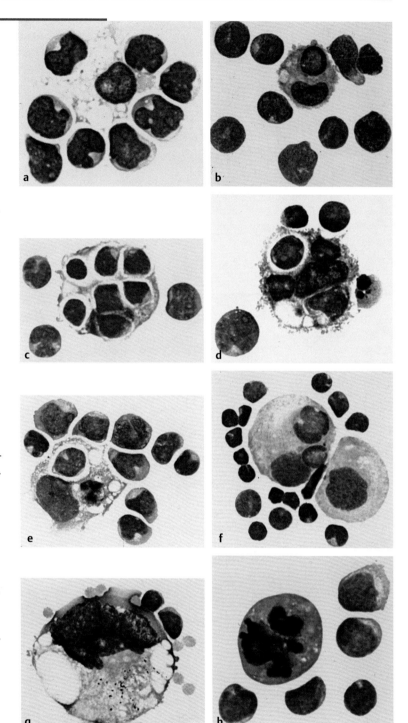

Fig. 5.**145** Small, chromatin-rich lymphoblasts containing little cytoplasm in a patient with CLL. The nuclei have multiple nucleoli; and a pathological mitosis in prophase is seen. There are also a few monocytes, some of which are activated. Note: cytological findings of this type are common in chronic leukemia and can be confused with those of viral meningitis, in which the activated lymphocytes have a similar appearance. Immunocytochemical marker tests should be done to establish the differential diagnosis whenever it is unclear.

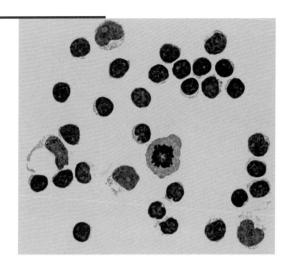

Fig. 5.**146** Leukemic meningitis in a patient with AML.
a Collection of uniform myeloblasts showing a tendency to mature into promyelocytes (FAB M2). The markedly basophilic cytoplasm has acidophilic, sometimes granulated perinuclear clearing in the Golgi zones and protuberances of the cell membrane.
b Myeloblasts in groups, some of them connected by cytoplasmic bridges, with the same characteristics as described above in a.

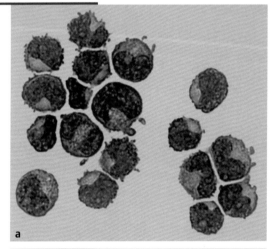

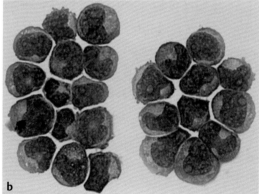

Fig. 5.**147** Large, loose cluster of mye-loblasts in a patient with acute mye-loid leukemia. The cells have a chro-matin-rich, hyperchromatic nucleus containing nucleoli and basophilic cytoplasm. In the center of the figure is a mitosis in prophase.

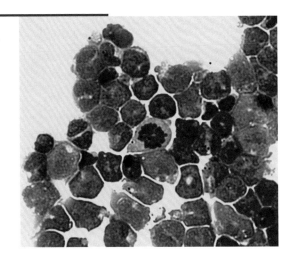

Fig. 5.**148** Leukemic meningitis in a patient with AML, displaying a marked tendency toward cell maturation. An erythroblast or myeloblast is seen in the top right corner. Next to it are myeloid blasts or myelocytes of vary-ing degrees of maturity, metamyelo-cytes, and degenerated cells.

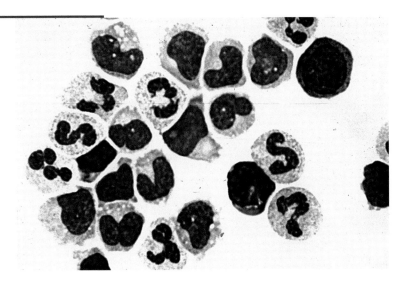

Fig. 5.**149** Myeloid blasts/myelocytes and neutrophilic granulocytes in a patient with AML. An apoptotic cell is seen in the top right of the figure.

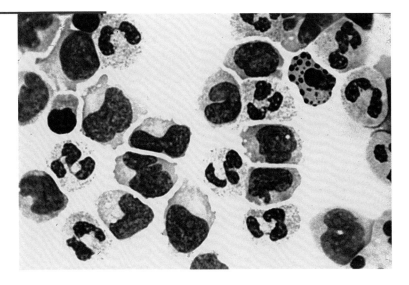

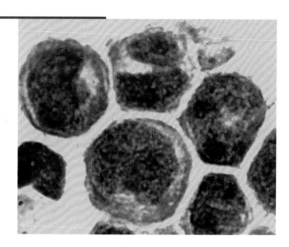

Fig. 5.**150** Monoblasts in a patient with *monocytic leukemia* (FAB M5). Features include hyperchromatic nucleus of variable ploidy with large nucleoli and markedly basophilic cytoplasm with perinuclear clearing.

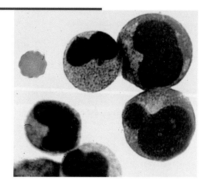

Fig. 5.**151** Leukemic meningitis in a patient with *monocytic leukemia* (FAB M5). Promonocytes in various stages of maturation: the nucleus has clearly visible nucleoli; the cytoplasm is basophilic, with acidophilic granules in some of the cells. The erythrocyte provides an indication of the scale.

Fig. 5.**152** Morphological comparison of leukemic blast forms in the CSF, blood, and bone marrow of a patient with a *chloroma* (subtype of acute myeloid leukemia). **a** Loose cell clusters in the CSF. **b** The corresponding peripheral blood smear. **c** Cell aggregates in autologous bone marrow.

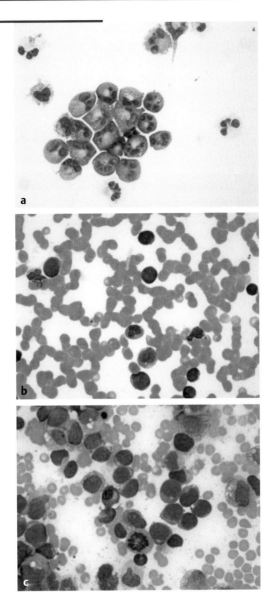

6 Pathological CSF Cell Findings in Cysts

V. Wieczorek, H. Kluge

The 1993 classification of the World Health Organization (WHO) still grouped cysts and tumorlike lesions together under a single heading that encompassed *Rathke cysts, epidermoid cysts, colloid cysts of the third ventricle*, and *nasal glioma* (nasal glial heterotopia). The current classification (2000) no longer counts the various types of central nervous system (CNS) cyst among tumors of the CNS. Nevertheless, we have included them in this atlas because they can shed cells of relatively characteristic types into the cerebrospinal fluid (CSF), which can occasionally be confused with tumor cells.

From the point of view of the CSF cytologist, the more important types of CNS cyst are epidermoid cysts (cholesteatoma) and dermoid cysts, as these can manifest themselves through *meningeal irritative forms* (reactive forms), as seen in Figures 6.1–6.5.

Epithelial cells can become trapped in the brain during development as the neural tube closes and later develop into a variety of lesions, most commonly dermoid and epidermoid cysts. Dermoid cysts can also arise from undifferentiated teratomas (see Chapter 5, Germ Cell Tumors) in which only the external germ cell layer differentiates into multilayered squamous epithelium and the other germ cell layers degenerate. Epidermoid cysts sometimes develop as the result of the iatrogenic transfer of clusters of epithelial cells into the intrathecal compartment, e.g., during neurosurgical procedures or lumbar puncture.

Dermoid cysts are lined with multiple layers of squamous epithelium; their walls can contain skin appendages (sebaceous and sweat glands) and even hair. Epidermoid cysts (cholesteatomas) are lined with multiple layers of keratinizing squamous epithelium. The degenerating cellular and tissue material (keratohyalin, keratinous debris, cholesterol esters) gradually accumulates, so that the cyst slowly expands like a tumor. Epidermoid cysts are not tumors in the strict sense of the term, however, because their enlargement is not due to actual autonomous growth.

The CSF may contain epitheliumlike cells or cell clusters that have exfoliated from cysts of these two types. Furthermore, if the cyst contents escape into the CSF, their constituent substances (especially cholesterol esters) can additionally induce aseptic meningitis.

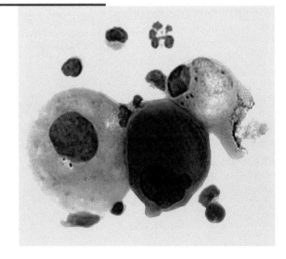

Fig. 6.1 Epitheliumlike cluster of large meningeal reactive cells in the CSF of a patient with an epidermoid cyst. The cells are in variable stages of activation, as indicated by the nuclear morphology (the nucleoli) and by variably intense acidophilia of the large cytoplasm. The middle cell shows marked poly- and hyperchromasia. The two other cells with looser cytoplasm have expelled fragments of nuclear chromatin.

Fig. 6.**2** Two meningeal reactive cells in a patient with an epidermoid cyst: large, peripherally located nucleus with nucleoli; copious, acidophilic cytoplasm with vacuolated protuberances from the intensely stained periphery (elimination of secretory products, after apparent ingestion and degradation of cyst contents?).

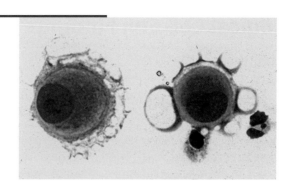

Fig. 6.**3** Meningeal reactive cell in a patient with an epidermoid cyst: eccentrically located nucleus; giant vacuole ("monstrous" signet-ring cell), with a more densely staining, acidophilic rim of cytoplasm. The vacuole probably contains material from a dermoid fistula, similar to the situation in the original cyst.

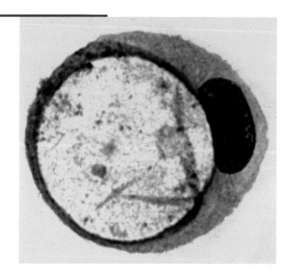

Fig. 6.**4** Very large reactive cells (one mononuclear, one binucleated) in a patient with an epidermoid cyst (reactive pleocytosis). The nuclei are coarsely structured and polyploid; the cytoplasm is acidophilic and coarsely or finely granulated. There are acinous, basophilic, fine and coarse vesicles attached to the cytoplasmic membrane. The associated, mildly misshapen granulocytes give an idea of the scale.

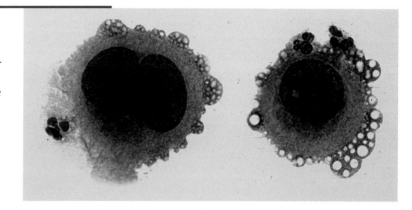

Fig. 6.**5** Multinucleated reactive cell in a patient with an epidermoid cyst showing poly- and hyperchromasia. The nuclei vary greatly in size and shape. The cytoplasm contains large vacuoles; its periphery is irregular with fine vesicles. A degenerated storage cell is seen on the right.

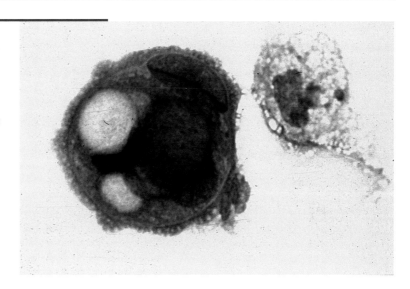

References

Aune MW, Becker JL, Bruguara C, et al. Automated flow cytometric analysis of blood cells in cerebrospinal fluid. *Am J Clin Pathol* 2004;121:690–700.

Cervos-Navarro J, Ferszt R (eds). *Klinische Neuropathologie*. Stuttgart: Thieme; 1989.

Den Hartog Joger WA. *Color Atlas of CSF: Cytopathology.* Lippincott: Philadelphia; 1980.

Dommasch D, Mertens HG (eds). *Cerebrospinalflüssigkeit – CSF.* Stuttgart: Thieme; 1980.

Dufresne JJ. *Cytologie pratique du liquide cephalorachidien.* Bâle: Ciba-Geigy SA; 1972.

Dux R, Faustmann PM, Lennartz K, Zimmermann CW. Durchflußzytometrische Liquorzelldiagnostik. *Acta Neurol* 1994;21:95–98.

Felgenhauer K, Beuche W (eds). *Labordiagnostik neurologischer Erkrankungen.* Stuttgart: Thieme; 1999.

Gandolfi A. The cytology of cerebral neuroblastoma, *Acta cytol* 1980;24:344–346.

Kleihues P, Cavenee WK (eds). *Pathology and Genetics of Tumours of the Nervous System.* Lyon: IARC Press; 2000.

Kleine TO, Hackler R, Mix E, Albrecht J, Kaiser C, Müller HAG. Analyse von Lymphozyten-Subpopulationen im Liquor cerebrospinalis. In: Schmitz G, Rothe G (eds). *Durchflußzytometrie in der klinischen Zelldiagnostik.* Stuttgart: Schattauer; 1994:189–197.

Kölmel HW. *Liquorzytologie.* Berlin: Springer; 1978.

Lehmitz R, Kleine TO. Liquorzytologie: Ausbeute, Verteilung und Darstellung von Leukozyten bei drei Sedimentationsverfahren im Vergleich zu drei Zytozentrifugen-Modifikationen. *Lab Med* 1994;18: 91–99.

Oehmischen M. *Cerebrospinal Fluid Cytology. An Introduction and Atlas.* Stuttgart: Thieme; 1976.

Oreja-Guevara C, Sindern E, Raulf-Heimsoth M, Malin JP. Analysis of lymphocyte subpopulations in cerebrospinal fluid and peripheral blood in patients with multiple sclerosis and inflammatory diseases of the nervous system. *Acta Neurol Scand* 1998;98: 310–313.

Pittenger MF, Mackay AM, Beck SC, et al. Mutilineage Potential of Adult Human Mesenchymal Stem Cells. *Science* 1999;284:143–147.

Radner H, Blümcke I, Reifenberger G, Wiestler OD. Die neue WHO-Klassifikation der Tumoren des Nervensystems 2000. Pathologie und Genetik. *Pathologe* 2002;23:260–283.

Schmidt RM. *Atlas der Liquorzytologie.* Leipzig: Barth; 1978.

Schmidt RM. *Der Liquor cerebrospinalis.* Leipzig: Thieme; 1987.

Sindern E. Role of Chemokines and their Receptors in the Pathogenesis of Multiple Sclerosis. *Frontiers in Bioscience* 2004;9:457–463.

Sindern E, Patzold T, Ossege LM, Gisevius A, Malin JP. Expression of chemokine receptor CXCR3 on cerebrospinal fluid T-cells is related to active MRI lesion appearance in patients with relapsing-remitting multiple sclerosis. *J Neuroimmunol* 2002;131: 186–190.

Stein H. Die neue WHO-Klassifikation der malignen Lymphome. *Pathologe* 2000;21:101–105.

Strik H, Luthe H, Nagel I, et al. Automated cerebrospinal fluid cytology. Limitations and reasonable applications. *Analyt Quant Cytol Histol* 2005;27: 167–173.

Thomas L (ed). *Labor und Diagnose.* Frankfurt/Main: TH-Books Verlagsgesellschaft; 1998.

Watson CW, Hajdu SI. Cytology of primary neoplasms of the central nervous system. *Acta cytol* 1977;21: 40–47.

Zettl UK, Lehmitz R, Mix E (eds). *Klinische Liquordiagnostik.* Berlin: Walter de Gruyter; 2003.

Historical References (Early Publications of the Jena School of CSF Cytology)

Greger J, Wieczorek V. Über das Vorkommen von Plasmazellen im Liquor cerebrospinalis bei neurologischen Erkrankungen. *Z Nervenheilk* 1956;23:366–374.

Sayk J. Ergebnisse neuer liquorcytologischer Untersuchungen mit dem Sedimentier-Kammerverfahren. *Ärztl. Wschr* 1954:1042.

Sayk J. *Cytologie der Cerebrospinalflüssigkeit.* Jena: Gustav Fischer; 1960.

Sayk J, Wieczorek V. Über besondere Verlaufsformen der Meningitis. Zur Frage der retothelialen Riesenzellmeningitis. *Arch Psychiat Nervenkr* 1960;200: 182–196.

Wieczorek V. Liquorveränderungen bei Blutungen in den Subarachnoidalraum mit besonderer Berücksichtigung des Liquorzellbildes. *Dtsch Z Nervenheilk* 1964a;186:87–100.

Wieczorek V. Erfahrungen mit der Tumorzelldiagnostik im Liquor cerebrospinalis bei primären und metastatischen Hirngeschwülsten. *Dtsch Z Nervenheilk* 1964b;186:410–432.

Wieczorek V. Wert und Grenzen der klassischen Liquorzelldiagnostik. *Lab Med* 1991;15:31–33.

Wieczorek V, Stahl J, Bock R. Zum Vorkommen von Riesenzellen in Liquor cerebrospinalis. *Dtsch Z Nervenheilk* 1967a;192:246–264.

Wieczorek V, Stahl J, Brodkorb W, Kluge H. Zum Vorkommen von Lymphoidzellen im Liquor cerebrospinalis. *Psychiat Neurol* 1967b;154:384–397.

Wieczorek V, Stahl J, Kluge H. Klinische und besonders tierexperimentielle Liquorzelluntersuchungen zur Genese von Riesenzellen im Liquor cerebrospinalis. *Dtsch Z Nervenheilk* 1968;194:296–310.

Wieczorek V, Zintl F, Stahl J, Aurich G. Liquorveränderungen bei der Meningeosis leucaemica. *Fol Haematol* 1971;5:357–365.

Wieczorek V, Waldmann K-D, Teweleit H-D, Hoffmeyer O. Melano-Phakomatose vom Typus der Melanoblastose neurocutanée Touraine unter Berücksichtigung der Liquorzytologie. *Dtsch Ges Wesen* 1972; 27:987–991.

Wieczorek V, Schmidt RM, Olischer R. Zur Standardisierung der Liquorzelldiagnostik. *Dtsch Ges Wesen* 1974;29:423–426.

Index

Page numbers in italics refer to figures.

A

acute lymphatic leukemia (ALL)   120, *121–123*
acute myelogenous leukemia (AML)   120–121, *124–126*
adenocarcinoma   63, 99
  breast   *100–102*
  cervix/uterus   *106, 107*
  colon   *104–105*
  gallbladder   *105*
  gastric   *103, 104*
  lung   *110–111*
AIDS (acquired immune deficiency syndrome)   25, 26
amitoses   63, *74, 118*
artifacts, lumbar puncture   13, 15, 18, *18–20*, 46
astrocytic tumors   64–66, *66–76*
astrocytomas
  anaplastic   65, *68*
  diffuse   65
  high-grade (grades III and IV)   65–66, *68–75*
  low-grade (grades I and II)   65, *66–67*
  pilocytic   64–65, *66*
  subependymal giant-cell   65
atypical cells   4, 65, *67, 79*
autoimmune diseases   26

B

bacterial infections   25, *27–31*
bacteriophage   47
basophilic granulocytes   21–22
B cell lymphoma   113–114, *114, 115*
B cells *see* B lymphocytes
bilirubin   45
bladder carcinoma   *112*
blast precursor cells   22
  leukemia   120–121, *121–127*
  malignant lymphoma   113, *114–118*
bloody CSF   7, 9, 45–46
B lymphocytes   4, 6, 13, 22
  activated *see* lymphocytes, activated
bone marrow cells   10, 18, *18, 19, 20*
brain abscess   *33*
breast carcinoma   99, *100–102*

bronchial carcinoma *see* lung carcinoma
Burkitt lymphoma   *117*

C

capillaries   18, *20*
carcinoembryonic antigen (CEA)   *105*
carcinoma cells   99–100
carcinomatous meningitis   61, 62, *70*, 99, *102*
cartilage cells   13, 18, *20*
CD20 antigen   *114*
cell membrane, tumor cells   63, *72, 78, 91*
cells
  damage   7, 8
  numbers required   4, 6
  preparation   8–9
centrifugation   5–6, 7, 8–9
centrocytic lymphoma   *115*
cerebral atrophy   46
cerebral infarction   47, *58*
cervical carcinoma   *106–107*
chloroma   113, 121, *127*
cholesteatoma (epidermoid cyst)   129, *129–131*
choroid plexus tumors   79, *79–80*
chronic lymphatic leukemia (CLL)   120, *124*
chronic myeloid leukemia (CML)   120, 121
colloid cysts of third ventricle   129
colon carcinoma   *104–105*
containers, CSF   7
craniopharyngioma   64
cryptococcosis   25, 26, *38*
cysts   129, *129–131*
  pineal   82, *82–83*
  teratoma-derived   94, *95*, 129
cytokeratin 18 (CK 18)   *101, 105*
cytoplasm, tumor cells   63, 65, *67, 69, 79–80*

D

dermoid cysts   94, *95*, 129

E

embryonal tumors   76, 84
encephalitis, HIV   26, *38*
encephalomalacia   *58*
endocytogenesis   63, *70, 93,* 99–100, *106, 109*
endothelial cells   15, *20*
eosinophilic granulocytes   21, *23,* 25–26, *28, 30, 33*
ependymal cells   15, *17,* 48, *48, 49*
ependymal tumors   76, *77–78*
ependymoblastoma   76, 84
ependymomas   76, *77–78*
   anaplastic   76, *77–78*
epidermoid cysts   129, *129–131*
epileptic seizures, generalized   46
epithelial cells   15–16, *16, 17,* 48, *50*
erythroblasts   *19, 125*
erythrocytes   10, 46
   immature/progenitor cells   18, *18, 19*
erythro-/hemosiderophages   *20,* 45, *51–52, 53, 54, 111*
erythrophages   *32,* 45, *48, 49–55, 56*
erythrophagocytosis   45, 46, *49–55*
Escherichia coli meningitis   *31*
esophageal carcinoma   *103*
ethmoidal carcinoma   *113*

F

FAB classification, leukemia   120
flow cytometry   5–6
foam cells *see* lipophages
foreign body reactions   26, 45
fungal infections   25, *38*

G

gallbladder carcinoma   99, *105–106*
gangliocytoma   81
ganglioglioma   81, *81*
gastric carcinoma   *103–104*
gastrointestinal tumors   99, *103–106*
German Society for the Diagnostic Study of the
   Cerebrospinal Fluid and Clinical Neurochemistry
   (DGLN)   1, 9–10
germ cell tumors   94, *94–95,* 99
germinoma   94
giant cell glioblastoma   65, 66, *72–75*
giant cells   26–27, 47, *50, 59,* 66
   Langhans   26, *41*
   neoplastic   26–27, *43–44, 63, 66, 70, 72–75, 80, 123*
   reactive   26, *39–43*
giant cell sarcoma   66, 89
gitter cells *see* lipophages
glial fibrillary acidic protein (GFAP)   64–65, 66, 76, 84,
   89

glioblastoma (glioblastoma multiforme)   65–66,
   70–75
gliomas   64–66, *66–76*
   malignant   65
   nasal   129
gliosarcoma   65, 66
granulocytes   21–23
   in infectious/inflammatory diseases   25, 26, *27–30,*
   32–35
   phagocytosed   45, *53*
granulocytic sarcoma (chloroma)   113, 121, *127*
gross cystic disease fluid protein 15 (GCDFP 15)   *101*

H

hematoidin   45, *55, 58*
hematomacrophages   45–46, *48–59*
hematopoietic cells   18, *18–20*
hemorrhage   2–3, 45–46, *48–58*
   subarachnoid *see* subarachnoid hemorrhage
   tumor-associated   62, *98, 111*
hemosiderin   45, 46, *51, 52, 53*
hemosiderophages   45, *57–58, 96, 99*
herpes simplex virus (HSV) meningitis   *33*
histiocytes   45, 47, *50*
histiocytoma, malignant fibrous   89, *93*
Hodgkin disease   114, *118*
human immunodeficiency virus (HIV) encephalopathy
   26, *38*
hydrocephalus   79, 82
hypernephroma   *43,* 99, *111–112*
hypoxic-ischemic brain injury   45–46

I

immunoblastic lymphoma   *117, 118*
immunocytochemical tumor markers   4, 62, 64–65,
   66, 114
immunocytological phenotyping techniques   4
infectious diseases   2, 21–44
inflammatory diseases   4, 21–44, *59*
intracranial hemorrhage *see* hemorrhage
ischemic brain damage   46

L

Langhans giant cells   26, *41*
Legionnaire's disease   25
leptomeningeal metastases   61, 62, 99
leptospirosis   25
leukemia   4, 10, 120–121, *121–127*
leukemic meningitis   62, 120, *121–126*
leukophages   45, *53, 54, 55, 123*
lipid staining   46, *58*

lipophages (foam cells)   46, 47–48, *50, 56, 58*

lipophagocytosis   *40, 43,* 45, 46, *50, 52, 54–56*

listeriosis   25, *29*

lumbar puncture   8
   artifacts   13, 15, 18, *18–20,* 46
   time since   7, 15

lung carcinoma   99, 100, *108–111*

Lyme disease (neuroborreliosis)   25, *32*

lymphoblastic lymphoma   *118*

lymphoblasts   120, *121–123, 124*

lymphocytes   6, 13–15, *14*
   activated   4, 9–10, 13, 14, *15,* 21–23, *23–24*
   in infectious/inflammatory disease   25, 26, *29–38*

lymphoid cells   13, 22

lymphoma, malignant   4, 10, 113–114, *114–118*
   metastatic extracerebral   113
   primary CNS   113, *114, 115, 117*

lymphomatous meningitis   62, 113, 114, *118*

lymphosarcoma   *118*

M

macrophages   3, 45–46, *48–59*
   cells transforming into   13, 16, *17,* 47–48, *48–50*
   multipotent   45, *53, 54, 55, 56*
   origins   47–48

malaria, cerebral   25

malignant fibrous histiocytoma   89, *93*

May–Grünwald–Giemsa stain   1, 2, 4, 9

medulloblastoma   84, *85–87*
   of the retina   84, *87*

megakaryoblasts   18, *19*

melanin   45, 96, *97–99*

melanoblastoma   96, *98*

melanocytic lesions, primary   89, 96

melanocytoma   96

melanoma   96, *96–99*

melanophages   96, *99*

melanophakomatosis of Touraine type   *97*

meningeal irritation   45, 129, *129–131*

meningeal tumors   62, 89

meningioma   64, 89
   anaplastic   89

meningitis
   bacterial   *23,* 25, *27–31*
   carcinomatous *see* carcinomatous meningitis
   cryptococcal   26, *38*
   eosinophilic   *30, 102*
   giant cell   *39*
   granulocytic   *33, 56*
   hemorrhagic   *54*
   leukemic   62, 120, *121–126*
   lymphomatous   62, 113, 114, *118*
   tuberculous   26, *30, 41*
   viral   26, *33–37*

meningococci   *27, 28*

meningoencephalitis   *32, 42*
   early summer (ESME)   26
   hemorrhagic   *32, 53, 54, 56, 59*
   viral   *34*

meningothelial tumors   89

mesenchymal, non-meningothelial tumors   89, *89–93*

mesenchymal origin, cells of   15, *17,* 47–48, *49, 50*

metabolic-toxic events, acute   46

metastases   4, 61, 99–100, *100–113*
   drop   62, 79, 84
   intracerebral   61, 99
   leptomeningeal   61, 62, 99

microglial cells   47

microphages   47

mitoses, pathological   63, *71, 80, 93, 102, 107, 117*

monoblasts   120, *126*

monocyte-macrophage system (MMS)   47

monocytes   13–15, *14, 24,* 47
   activated   14, *15,* 22, *23, 24,* 45
   in hemorrhage   45, *48, 52*
   immature/progenitor cells   18, *20*
   in infectious/inflammatory disease   25, 26, *27–33, 36–38*

monocytic leukemia   *126*

mononuclear cells   5
   in hemorrhage and brain injury   45, *53, 57*
   in infectious/inflammatory diseases   25, *28, 29–38*

mononuclear phagocytic system (MPS)   47

"mulberry cell"   *35, 37*

multiple sclerosis (MS)   6

mumps meningitis   *35, 36*

Mycoplasma pneumoniae   25

myeloblasts   *18,* 120–121, *124–125*

myelocytes   *18, 19, 125*

myeloma, multiple   114

myelopoietic cells   18, *18, 19*

myelosarcoma *see* chloroma

N

nasal glioma   129

neoplastic cells *see* tumor cells

neurinoma   64

neuroblastoma   64, 84

neuroborreliosis   25, *32*

neurobrucellosis   25

neurocysticercosis   25–26

neurofilament protein   84

neuropathology, tumor   62

neutrophilic granulocytes   3, *18,* 21, *23,* 25, *27,* 47

non-Hodgkin lymphoma   *116*

normoblasts   18, *19*

nuclear-to-cytoplasmic ratio   63, 76, 84, *86, 87,* 99, 113–114

nuclei, tumor cells   63

nucleoli, tumor cells   63, *95, 111*

O

oligodendroglioma, anaplastic   64
opportunistic infections   25, 26
osteogenic sarcoma   89, *93*

P

Pappenheim stain *see* May–Grünwald–Giemsa stain
parasitic infections   25–26
pericytes   47–48
phagocytes   25, *29, 30*
phagocytosis   *27, 28, 30*
pH buffering   7
pineal cysts   82, *82–83*
pineal tumors   82, *82–84*
pineoblastoma (pinealoblastoma)   82
pineocytoma (pinealocytoma, pinealoma)   82, *83–84*
  anisomorphic   82, *83*
pituitary adenoma   88, *88*
pituitary carcinoma   88
plasmablastic sarcoma   114
plasma cells   9–10, 13, *20, 59*
  in infectious/inflammatory diseases   22–23, *24, 34–37*
  neoplastic   114, *119*
plasmacytoma   *92,* 113, *119*
pleocytosis
  granulocytic   25, *28,* 46
  reactive   26, *32, 33, 43, 45, 55, 56,* 62
plexus epithelial cells   15, *16*
polypropylene test tubes   7
primitive neuroectodermal tumor (PNET)   84
promonocytes   *126*
promyelocytes   *18, 19*
prostate carcinoma   100
protein additives   9
protozoal infections   25

R

Rathke cysts   129
renal cell carcinoma *see* hypernephroma
reporting form, CSF cytology   9–10, *11*
respiratory tract carcinoma   99, 100, *108–111*
reticular cells   47
reticulo-endothelial system (RES)   47
retinoblastoma   84, *87*
round-robin CSF cytology tests   1, 9, *11*
rubella   3*7*

S

sarcoma
  giant cell   66, 89
  granulocytic (chloroma)   113, 121, *127*
  meningeal   *44,* 89, *89–92*
  osteogenic   89, *93*
  plasmablastic   114
scavenger cells *see* lipophages
sedimentation, cell   7, *8–9*
  Sayk method   1, 7, 8
  see also centrifugation
seminoma, metastatic   94, *95*
siderophagocytosis   *55*
signet-ring cells   *43,* 46, *59,* 63
  epidermoid cyst-related   *130*
  metastatic carcinoma   99, *100, 103, 104, 105, 106*
  primary CNS tumors   *66, 69, 72, 93, 98*
skin cells   13, 18
small-cell carcinoma, lung   100, *108, 109*
specimen handling   7–8
spherocytes   21, *28, 54, 56*
spongioblastoma
  polar   65
  primitive polar   65, *75–76*
squamous-cell carcinoma   100
staining   9
subarachnoid hemorrhage   *17, 20,* 46, *48, 48–58*
subependymoma   76
surface epithelium cells   10, 13, 15–16, *16, 17*
synaptophysin   84
syphilis   25, *31*

T

T cell lymphoma   114
T cells *see* T lymphocytes
temperature, CSF storage   7
teratoma   94, *94, 95,* 129
T lymphocytes   6, 13
toxoplasmosis   25, 26, *38*
traumatic brain injury   45–46, *56, 57*
tuberculosis   25, 26, *30, 41*
tumor cells   3, 10, 61–64
  cannibalism *see* endocytogenesis
  diagnostic criteria   62–64
  exfoliation and migration into CSF   61
  giant *see* giant cells, neoplastic
  phagocytosed   45, *55*
tumor markers *see* immunocytochemical tumor markers
tumors   4, 61–119
  metastatic *see* metastases
  primary brain   61, 62, 64
  secondary brain   64
  WHO classification scheme   62, 63–64, 65, 129
tumor-suspect cells   4, 10, 61, 62–63, 64, *67, 112*

U

uterine carcinoma   *106–107*

V

varicella-zoster virus (VZV) meningitis   *34, 36*
ventricular CSF   3, *7–8*, 13, 16, 26, *33*, 46
ventriculitis   *33, 59*
vimentin   66, 89
viral infections   26, *33–37*
volume, CSF   *8–9*

W

Whipple disease   25
World Health Organization (WHO), tumor classification
    scheme   62, *63–64*, 65, 129

X

xanthoastrocytoma, pleomorphic   65, 66

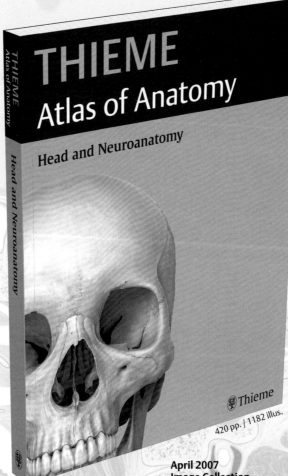
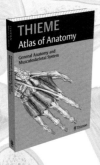
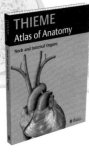
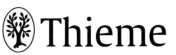